Marvels of Medicine

Literature and Scientific Enquiry in Early Colonial Spanish America

Liverpool Latin American Studies

Series Editor: Matthew Brown, University of Bristol
Emeritus Series Editor: Professor John Fisher

4 Bourbon Peru, 1750–1824
John Fisher

5 Between Resistance and Adaptation: Indigenous Peoples and the Colonisation of the Chocó, 1510–1753
Caroline A. Williams

6 Shining Path: Guerilla War in Peru's Northern Highlands, 1980–1997
Lewis Taylor

7 South American Independence: Gender, Politics, Text
Catherine Davies, Claire Brewster and Hilary Owen

8 Adventuring Through Spanish Colonies: Simón Bolívar, Foreign Mercenaries and the Birth of New Nations
Matthew Brown

9 British Trade with Spanish America, 1763–1808
Adrian J. Pearce

10 Colonial Tropes and Postcolonial Tricks: Rewriting the Tropics in the novela de la selva
Lesley Wylie

11 Argentina's Partisan Past: Nationalism and the Politics of History
Michael Goebel

12 The Reinvention of Mexico: National Ideology in a Neoliberal Era
Gavin O'Toole

13 Armies, Politics and Revolution: Chile, 1808–1826
Juan Luis Ossa Santa Cruz

14 Andean Truths: Transitional Justice, Ethnicity, and Cultural Production in Post-Shining Path Peru
Anne Lambright

15 Positivism, Science, and 'The Scientists' in Porfirian Mexico: A Reappraisal
Natalia Priego

16 Argentine Cinema and National Identity (1966–1976)
Carolina Rocha

17 Decadent Modernity: Civilization and 'Latinidad' in Spanish America, 1880–1920
Michela Coletta

18 Borges, Desire, and Sex
Ariel de la Fuente

19 Contacts, Collisions and Relationships: Britons and Chileans in the Independence era, 1806–1831
Andrés Baeza Ruz

20 Writing and the Revolution: Venezuelan Metafiction 2004–2012
Katie Brown

Liverpool Latin American Studies, New Series 21

Marvels of Medicine

Literature and Scientific Enquiry in Early Colonial Spanish America

Yarí Pérez Marín

LIVERPOOL UNIVERSITY PRESS

First published 2020 by
Liverpool University Press
4 Cambridge Street
Liverpool
L69 7ZU

British Library Cataloguing-in-Publication data
A British Library CIP record is available

ISBN 978 1 78962 250 8

Typeset by Carnegie Book Production, Lancaster
Printed and bound by CPI Group (UK) Ltd, Croydon CR0 4YY

Figures

Acknowledgements

Summers were a bit of a scramble for postgraduate students in my cohort back in the day, before offers in the humanities at my institution were restructured and new measures adopted. Funding, which was linked to undergraduate teaching, would run out in May and the choice of temporary jobs to carry you over until the start of the next academic year was usually not very appealing. In the hopes of avoiding a second stint teaching 'recreational' Spanish to the owner of a plastics company and his wife, the latter having warned me that she might need to let me go if I did not change my mind about homework assignments, I sent an unsolicited email to Norman Fiering, then Director of the John Carter Brown Library, whom I had met briefly during a class outing organised by Stephanie Merrim for the students in her colonial Latin American literature seminar. In that message I asked if there was anything—anything at all—that they would consider hiring me to do. A few months later, gratefully at work in a newly created position as ad hoc assistant to the library's staff, and charged among other things with physically organising new acquisitions so they would be ready for use by cataloguers, I came across a passage in one of these texts that was different from anything I had read up to that point in my training. It was a detailed explanation of how a child was conceived inside a mother's womb, of how the tiny parts of its body began to sprout and develop, with different structures growing and changing in appearance until it was ready to receive its soul, the timing of which varied depending on whether it was a boy or a girl, or one of the other categories it adduced.

What stopped me in my tracks then were not the questions that would come later: how was it possible to peer into a living human body in this way, sequentially and over an extended period? (Was it?) To what extent was the passage derived from the first-hand dissection of a dead body, as the source claimed, and how much was instead a kind of *Aristotle Redux*, with old ideas in new robes for readers in a 'new' world? Where did sensory observation end and, to borrow Inca Garcilaso's phrasing, where did the telltale European projection of desire that 'only saw what it wished to see' begin? And how did the other developmental possibilities given map onto emerging ideas on sex and gender? How unusual was this author's take? How unusual was *he* in the context of sixteenth century Mexican medicine? No. Instead, what drew me to want to know more about the book was its choice of language, the similes to be precise, for according to Alonso López de Hinojosos, the manner in which a baby was formed was very much like making a 'cuajada' (custard desert). To help readers see in their mind's eye the sizes, colours and textures of the structures he described the comparisons volunteered were to simmering liquids, jugs of milk, breadcrumbs, cochineal powder and garbanzo beans. Sor Juana was right, I thought: these were the 'philosophies of the kitchen' at play, in a surgical manual, anchoring the prose of an author who did seem a better writer for knowing how to cook.

From the experience that summer working as a temporary member of staff at the JCB, and thanks in no small part to Merrim's thoughtful guidance as my doctoral dissertation advisor as well as the support of José 'Pepe' Amor y Vázquez†, mentor extraordinaire, the seeds of this project were sown. The chance to be a part of two interdisciplinary initiatives in the years that followed would also prove key. The first was a spring seminar convened by Paula Findlen at the Folger Shakespeare Library focused on science, gender and knowledge in early modern Europe; the second was a year-long Pembroke Center research seminar organised by Anne Fausto-Sterling exploring the link between biology, social policy and theories of embodiment. The conversations I participated in at these two fora definitively changed my approach to the subject matter discussed in this book, if not to my fields of study more broadly.

I am indebted to many colleagues who became part of the writing process in one way or another. From reading an early draft and providing feedback, to including me in a conference panel or a publication that refined my thinking around an issue, to asking a timely question that warranted a better answer, to helping me find my way in a new city and its collections, even to sharing an offhand remark that ignited a spark, how fortunate am I to have benefitted from all of these gestures. Sacramento Roselló-Martínez, Lisa Voigt, Andrew Beresford, Andrea Noble†, Leigh Mercer, Santiago Fouz-Hernández, Nathalie Bouzaglo, Jorge Coronado, Lucille Kerr, Emily Maguire, Alejandra Uslenghi, Richard Gordon, Laura E. Matthew, Kerstin Oloff, F.-J. Hernández Adrián, Valentina Velázquez Zvierkova, Álvaro Álvarez Delgado, Pedro Pereira, Fermín del Pino, R. Jovita Baber, Michelle Molina, Domingo Ledezma, Rebecca Ferreboeuf, Dániel Margócsy, Óscar Fernández, Adam Miyashiro, Fiona Clark, Ken Ward, Ernesto Sierra, Deborah Taylor-Pearce, José Santos Guzmán, David Schoenbrun, María del Pilar Blanco, Anja-Silvia Goeing, Ken Alder, Elaine Leong, Manuel Hijano, Antonio Carreño, Mercedes López-Baralt, Patricia Oliart, Beatriz Cruz Sotomayor, Patience Schell and Marie-Claire Barnet: the traces of your intellectual generosity shine brightly in the pages ahead.

Institutional support has been key in providing the resources and the time away from teaching needed to undertake the kind of international and cross-disciplinary research that my analysis is built on and to bring the project to completion. Without the encouragement and funding of the Andrew W. Mellon Foundation Career Enhancement Fellowship, the Center for New World Comparative Studies Fellowship at the John Carter Brown Library and Durham University's Research Leave this book would not exist. Thanks are due also to Jonathan Long and the School of Modern Languages and Cultures at Durham University for their help with securing images and permissions.

I must acknowledge the helpfulness of members of staff at the John Carter Brown Library, the Folger Shakespeare Library, the British Library, the Huntington Library, the Biblioteca Nacional de España and the Bibliothèque nationale de France. I am particularly appreciative of the assistance received from Carmen Morales Mateo at the Biblioteca de Castilla-La Mancha, Stephen Greenberg at the US National Library of Medicine, History of Medicine Division, Jorge Juárez and María del Perpetuo Socorro Villarreal Escárrega at the Instituto Nacional de Antropología e Historia in Mexico, and Guadalupe Rodríguez at the Museo Nacional de Historia in Mexico.

My heartfelt thanks also to Chloé Johnson at Liverpool University Press for her acuity and her interest in the manuscript from the start, as well as to the two anonymous readers whose questions and good suggestions helped to give *Marvels of Medicine* its final shape. 'Impressive' seems woefully inadequate to describe the work of Rachel Chamberlain and her team at Carnegie Publishing, and their exemplary care in putting this book together in the midst of a global pandemic.

To Yoko Clarke, Elizabeth and Gina Collings, José Luis Pabón and Christian Mieves, whose assistance has been invaluable in helping me navigate the challenges of a transatlantic life over the past few years: thank you. And to Carmen Pérez Marín, Edwin Seda Fernández, Zagra (Tita) Pérez Anazagasty† and Lucía Seda, my debts are too numerous and too great to list here. Far more than a mere book has been made possible only because of your long-standing and unwavering support.

Marvels of Medicine is dedicated to my parents, E. Ferdinand Pérez Anazagasty† and Ivette Marín Cancel.

Introduction

Medical books and colonial Latin American literature

One of the challenges when speaking about colonial Latin American literature as a concept is that it asks us to first concede it exists. Even before we can come to an agreement as to the kinds of texts it would describe—oral, written, performative—, we are confronted with an identity rubric that invokes a series of 'imagined communities'[1] known to be exclusionary and incomplete. Each one of its components—colonial, Latin American, literature—places us in contested and politicised terrain, and the use of the label ratifies the combining of competing political agendas under one seemingly common project, arbitrarily compartmentalised along socio-linguistic lines. The phrase privileges a teleological association between Europe and ancient Rome at the expense of a number of other possible (although admittedly equally incomplete) contenders, given the region's diverse cultural and ethnic composition. It makes geographic contiguity into an unconvincing assertion on cultural cohesion for a historical period during which the cities of Mexico and Cuzco had far more in common with places in the Pacific like Goa or Manila than they did with the not-yet-founded European settlements of the South American River Plate. It also claims literariness for a host of historiographical materials (ships' logs, letters, autobiographical accounts, philosophical treatises) that scholars, depending on their understanding of literature as a genre, do not all see as possessing the qualities that would allow them to be defined as such. Assailed on multiple fronts, the study of colonial Latin American literature retreats into the safety of structure in modern language departments where the academic study of Iberian and Ibero-American culture has come to be organised predominantly around time

1 A concept put forth by Benedict Anderson in 1983 that understood nationalism as a social construct of the late colonial period. Anderson argued that the ability of individuals from the same region to converge upon a common definitional imaginary, despite socio-economic differences and the absence of direct contact, became a key factor enabling the consolidation of modern nations. Anderson's framework has since been used to theorise other kinds of networks and communities, before and beyond the rise of the nation.

and sequence. There it gambles on the illusion that the temporal proximity to the epic or the *chanson de geste* on the one hand, and to the masterworks of Golden Age theatre and prose fiction on the other, will shield it from having to make a case on its own, as literature, or be asked to account for its vast archive of materials composed prior to 1816,[2] before as well as after 1492, that do not fall neatly within the purview of either lyric or drama. The distinctive hybridity that would have this corpus stand out in the larger stage of world literature is toned down or partially disavowed, freeing it to be engaged by questions in a number of disciplines perhaps but at the expense of having its literariness pass for a dead metaphor.

Writing on colonial studies more broadly (not just literature), Yolanda Martínez-San Miguel has explained that substituting 'early modern' for 'colonial' in order to describe it as an interdisciplinary field, far from resolving the issue, brings its own set of associations, organising time and measuring development along a Western solipsism (2008, 25). In a project such as this one, which focuses on the medical and surgical print outputs of what was in sixteenth-century Mexico and the Caribbean a politically dominant yet demographically tiny community of the sum total of the region's inhabitants, describing imprints from the period as 'colonial Latin American texts' would make it seem as if their authors were expressing assurances about a future they could not have imagined, let alone would have chosen to envision along those lines. Yet despite the presentist obstacle arising from this dissonance, Martínez-San Miguel argues for the usefulness of retaining 'colonial' less as a position on identity, or one claiming to speak for entities that are not necessarily represented in that utterance, and more as a tool that concentrates the discussion on a study of power relationships between metropolitan centres and peripheries which are often (although not exclusively) demarcated along European versus non-European geographic spaces. This distinction enables us not only to keep colonial on the table, but helps to show why it is a crucial framework with which to analyse medical books written in the sixteenth century in, or about, what would eventually come to be known as Latin America.

Most of the period imprints that comprise the colonial Latin American literature canon for the sixteenth century are not objects from the region per se, at least not in a literal sense. In a story of expanding empires, a lack of correspondence between the place where a work was written and where it was published, or between the geographic location it describes and the author's own background or place of residence, is hardly unusual and often an imperative. Bartolomé de Las Casas's *Brevísima relación de la destruición de las Indias* [An account, much abbreviated, of the destruction of the Indies] (1552) arguably had to be printed with Sevillian ink given what it sought to

2 Composition date of José Joaquín Fernández de Lizardi's *El periquillo sarniento* (Mexico 1816), generally considered the first novel to be written and published in Latin America.

do and who it wanted to reach.[3] Likewise, there are contextual reasons for why the pages of Álvar Núñez Cabeza de Vaca's *Relación y comentarios* [The account of Alvar Nuñez Cabeza de Vaca] (1555) or Gonzalo Fernández de Oviedo's *Libro XX de la segunda parte de la general historia de las Indias* [Book XX of the Second Part of the General History of the Indies] (1557) both see the light of day in Francisco Fernández de Córdoba's shop in Valladolid and not in New Spain.[4] But how, then, do we justify not placing a text like Pedro Arias de Benavides's *Secretos de Chirurgia* [Secrets of Surgery] (1567) in their company, being as it was, printed by the same man, likely sown together by the same sets of hands, with page upon page narrating events and first-hand experiences that had transpired in the same part of the world, and at times going over very similar subject matter? Are the first two literary in a way the third one is not? By extension, on what basis do we exclude from consideration almost all of the 131[5] surviving texts printed in Mexico in the sixteenth century from the remit of colonial literature? Is there a clear set of criteria at work that decides they are any less fit for consideration in early modern literary studies than the voyage accounts, *historias*, letters, *relaciones*, and moral treatises that shape the colonial Latin American literature canon at present? What is gained or lost by having locally produced texts like these be thought of as the exclusive domain of historians, linguists and cultural studies scholars but not scholars of literature?

In Rosa María Fernández de Zamora's bibliography of New Spain's sixteenth-century imprints, the most complete list available to date and one that updates considerably Joaquín García Icazbalceta's, she places only two titles in the category of 'Literature and Theater' (2009, 357). The rest are described as religious manuals, sermons, dictionaries, theological treatises, instructions for tax collectors, and so on. Others are harder to pin down: a book on arithmetic pertaining to the gold and silver mines of Peru, several works on funeral rites, one on the art of war, a couple on Aristotelian philosophy, some on emblems, quite a few on the lives of saints. Considered as a

3 The titles of period works in Latin or Spanish are provided as originally written, with subsequent mentions shortened for ease, except in the case of Monardes's *Historia medicinal* which will be referred to as such given the range of variation in how the work was known in the sixteenth century. Spelling has been modernised in transcriptions from the texts themselves, including cases where quotes are taken from a modern edition. Lexical archaisms are generally allowed to remain if they do not obscure meaning. Unless otherwise specified, translations into English are my own.

4 See Alcocer y Martínez (1926). The first 19 books of what came to be known as the *Historia general y natural de las Indias* [General and natural history of the Indies] were published in 1535, and the first book of the second part in 1552. The complete version of the *Historia* would not be published until the nineteenth century.

5 Approximately 220 are believed to have been printed in Mexico between 1539 and 1600, with 136 surviving (four were published in 1600). This calculation follows the most current information in Fernández de Zamora as well as in the Primeros Libros digital portal.

group, although the majority appeared in either Spanish or Latin, 47 of those that survive were written at least partly in an Indigenous language. Texts printed not just in Nahuatl but in P'urhepecha, Huasteco, Mixtec, Zapotec languages, Otomi, Chocho, Tzotzil, all passed through the wooden beds of colonial Mexican printing presses in the sixteenth century. Excising these works from the repertoire of Latin American literary history on the basis of an assumed consensus about their non-literary status effectively closes the door on the possibility that they would have something valuable to contribute if read through that disciplinary framework. When we do take the time to examine many of these texts with the tools of literary analysis alongside those of history and cultural studies, a wealth of information emerges on the sensibilities and mores of colonial subjects. Even in works seemingly devoid of narrative, frequently there are prefaces explaining to period readers their context and purpose in which can be found strategies and tropes not unlike those of the *relación* or early modern *historias*.

As with inquisitorial censorship practices, where the crossing out of a line only makes it shine brightly for future readers empowered by newer technologies, the warnings and prohibitions in texts like church ordinances reveal otherwise missed nuances when one attempts to see them through the eyes of the period listeners who increasingly witnessed similar behaviours either denounced or celebrated for their entertainment in poems and *romances*, as well as on stage. Consider, for instance, the multiple readings that emerge from a text such as the *Constituciones del arçobispado y provincia dela muy ynsigne y muy leal ciudad de Tenuxtitlan Mexico dela nueua España* [Ordinances of the archbishopric and province of the very illustrious and loyal city of Tenochtitlan-Mexico of New Spain] (1556). At face value, its list of instructions is a formidable display of the Church's power over the public and private lives of individuals. But if one reads between the lines, its repetitiveness, circumlocution and emphasis on the most minute of details when it turns to the policing of ongoing transgressions ultimately betrays sentiments of consternation and impotence. In addition, the ample space afforded to the denunciation of what it sees as aberrant practices also lets us glimpse otherwise invisible and inaccessible expressions of popular will in the colonial record, marked by irreverence, practicality and even a sense of humour: Indigenous people should not be allowed to take home holy water or chrism for private use, and priests are advised to place these under lock and key (fol. 18r); Spaniards are reminded they should not skip mass on Sundays to host banquets, or drink in taverns or make public noise thereby 'scandalising the newly converted Indians who see them thus', and generally 'setting a bad example' (fol. 12r); Spaniards in possession of enslaved Africans are reminded that they need to set time aside for them to attend mass and not put them to work on feast days lest owners 'be rigorously punished' (fol. 12v); card games, ball games, sleeping and dancing are all prohibited in churches and cemeteries (fol. 16r); 'the fidelity of marriage ... is perverted by the practice many adopt of publicly parading their mistresses' and both the man and the mistress shall henceforth be punished 'with excommunication, ipso facto' (fol. 22r); priests are forbidden from 'wearing red, or yellow, or green or light blue' (fol. 25r), as well as from 'dancing, singing … watching bullfights or [participating in] other dishonest spectacles' (fol. 25v); while it is understandable that priests will experience stress and moments of frustration, they should refrain from taking in vain 'the name of God, or Our Lady, or the saints' or uttering 'God be damned, or Holy Mary, or I do not believe in Him, or other similar blasphemies', and 'if any religious official is seen performing these actions, regardless of his station', he is to pay 20 pesos 'per instance' (fol. 25v); priests are also reminded that they are not to have concubines 'either inside or outside the home', and 'if at present they should have them, they are hereby advised to end their association within 30 days' (fol. 26v). As it pertains to medicine specifically, the *Constituciones* offer the following:

> We command that the doctors in our archbishopric and province who are called upon to cure, that on their first visit they instruct and coax patients, regardless of their status, wealth or condition, to confess their sins and put their souls in order … and if the aforementioned patient does not do as told, and the doctor finds out that he has not confessed, he is to refuse to visit him a second time, and should not dispense any medicine for his health until he truly and sincerely confesses and takes communion and puts his soul in order … and so that this comes to be known by all we command that the priests read these instructions in church the first four Sundays of lent.[6]

Over the years I spent conducting the research I now share in this book I became increasingly persuaded that the reasons why medical texts tended to remain always just outside the scope of my training as a literature scholar were teleological rather than historical, or even disciplinary. Whether or not I accepted the late fifteenth century and the arrival of Europeans as a foundational moment in the history of Latin America, I was still part of a cultural and scholarly community that suppressed caveats when it came to finding points of contact with the writings of figures like Christopher

6 'Mandamos a los médicos de nuestro arzobispado y provincia que fueren llamados a curar, que luego en la primera visitación amonesten e induzcan a los enfermos, de cualquier estado, preeminencia o condición que sean: que se confiesen y ordenen sus ánimas … Y si el tal enfermo no lo hiciere así, el médico después que supiere que el enfermo no se ha confesado, no lo vaya a visitar la segunda vez ni les recete cosa alguna para su salud: hasta que realmente y con efecto se confiesen y comulguen y ordenen su ánima … porque venga esto a noticia de todos mandamos que los primeros cuatro domingos de cuaresma los curas publiquen esta constitución en sus iglesias' (fols. 7v–8r). I have translated the instructions assuming a male patient, since the text uses 'el enfermo', but there is no indication that women would be exempt from the same directive in this instance. The phrasing also weaves in and out of the plural and the singular.

Columbus or Bernal Díaz del Castillo, however problematic these could be when taken as canonical sources by Latin Americanists, but balked at the thought of tracing the origins of this literary tradition to a set of conversion manuals, or bureaucratic Church edicts, Spanish-to-Nahuatl dictionaries, or to books on stomach problems and broken bones. To a certain degree, I was one of Michael Solomon's 'literary historians, preoccupied with the singular genius of writers such as Rojas, Garcilaso, Quevedo, and Góngora, [who] resisted examining the rhetorical and narrative elements in works primarily identified as guidebooks and instruction manuals [like] vernacular medical writing' (2010, 3–4), a task seemingly best left to bibliographers, linguists and religious scholars.

The doctors and surgeons who came to the Americas were, in many ways, no different than other would-be emissaries of European value systems, cultures, languages and social institutions. Writing on events transpiring outside Europe, they began to make Europeanness itself a site from which to claim legitimacy over other possible sites of enunciation, thus bolstering the importance of emerging notions on matters like identity and race within a process then still strongly conditioned by wealth, social, political or religious standing, patronage, gender and, to a lesser degree, education. Their assertion that something was true and known 'por experiencia', that its ontological reality could be vouched for by the individual and his or her definition of direct contact, is a commonplace claim in sixteenth-century European science and medicine, and a phrase that recurs in many materials unrelated to the Americas or the colonial experience. And yet, as is well known, the notion of authority being conferred by way of witnessing is a core epistemological gesture in the texts that make up the early colonial Latin American canon. As men who had all been born in Europe to later set sail for the Americas, the four medical practitioners I focus on in this book—Pedro Arias de Benavides, Alonso López de Hinojosos, Agustín Farfán and Juan de Cárdenas—all saw themselves (at least initially) as voices within a larger conversation on health and the human body, one driven by their trust in the merits of combining scholarly rigour with personal experience. But in the process of becoming authors (and as I argue, New World authors in particular, every one), they found themselves contesting the supremacy of emerging marginalising colonial structures not on the grounds of birthright, as *criollos* would do later on, but of science. Their texts crystallise a unique moment in the history of Latin American culture because they stood at the intersection of medicine and coloniality, turning to the literary experience in an effort to maintain that ultimately untenable position; *Marvels of Medicine* is first and foremost an attempt to tell this story and to critically unpack its significance.

A note of caution, though. The chapters that follow do not seek to make medical texts into something they are not, nor do they share the romanticised view of many of the great twentieth-century Latin American artists, poets and filmmakers who mined the colonial past for inspiration, speaking about chroniclers as would-be novelists, or of the present as prophecy come to fruition. As valuable and productive as those endeavours have been, ours has a different set of objectives. Instead, the case studies I bring forward aim to reconstruct the kinds of readings that would have been possible during the sixteenth and early seventeenth centuries based on the simple yet cardinal observation that the majority of colonial subjects who interacted with textual sources at this time did so not as writers but as readers, with reading as a social practice that would be key to the formation of colonial Latin America. Although admittedly overshadowed by the level of production in places like Frankfurt or Venice, still, the output of print materials in Mexico City would surpass that of many other cities of the sixteenth century with access to comparable print technology, whether in Europe or in contact zones. As Fernández de Zamora puts it:

> Valladolid, which at times served as the capital of Castile, produced 371 titles; Toledo, which was a capital city under Charles V, printed 439; Cordoba, which had enjoyed great prominence under Arab dominion, was not able to sustain it, printing only 51 works; and what can be said of Segovia, which printed only 11 titles … in Lima, Peru, 18 titles were printed; in the Asian cities of Goa, where the printing press arrived in 1557, and in the cities of Manila, Macau, Katsusa, Makusa and Nagasaki, where it arrived later, the total output of the presses did not exceed 40 titles total. (2009, 46)

In comparison, 'the city of Mexico-Tenochtitlan, fresh out of a war of conquest and with a still scarce reading public, produced around 300 printed books, booklets and broadsheets' (Fernández de Zamora, 2009, 46). In addition to circulating manuscripts and print sources, readers in the New World were also avid consumers of imported volumes. As Irving Leonard remarked in his study on the Mexican book trade of 1576, '[i]n view of the relatively small number of Europeans in the viceroyalty of New Spain, the quantities of books imported were remarkably large, and the booksellers surprisingly numerous', further observing that among the imports dealing with science, medicine was the preferred subject (1992, 199, 201). Health and illness were central preoccupations for the people of early colonial Mexico who had witnessed frequent and widespread epidemics of smallpox and *cocoliztli* (often rendered in Spanish as *cocoliste* or *cocolistle*, meaning 'great pestilence' in Nahuatl) that had decimated Indigenous populations. New Spain suffered at least 15 serious epidemics during the sixteenth century. At the same time, its inhabitants had to contend with daily non-lethal aliments, from severe to mild, as evidenced in the frequency with which they are mentioned not only in medical literature proper, but in travel accounts, chronicles, letters and various kinds of documents.

Situating books on medicine and surgery in a context that is sensitive to setting and interpersonal connections can expand our understanding of medical authors as part of a literary sector in the early colonial world.

Writers of scientific, philosophical and more narrowly defined literary works alike shared the common experience of being readers themselves, raising new questions about the extent to which this informed their craft when it came to setting down on paper their own thoughts and ideas, and to try to capture the attention of others. As Michel Foucault reminds us in the case of Ulisse Aldrovandi, the sixteenth-century Italian naturalist considered by some the 'father of modern natural history', the scientific prose of the period could be 'an inextricable mixture of exact descriptions, reported quotations, fables without commentary, remarks dealing indifferently with an animal's anatomy, its use in heraldry, its habitat, its mythological values, or uses to which it could be put in medicine or magic' (2005, 43). The scope and variety of information in sixteenth-century texts would lead later naturalists from the eighteenth century, like Georges-Louis Leclerc, Comte de Buffon, to question the percentage of writing that actually concerned what he would have deemed science. Cited by Foucault, and referring to a passage by Aldrovandi, Buffon declares: '"Let it be judged after that what proportion of natural history is to be found in such a hotch-potch of writing. There is no description here, only legend." And indeed, for Aldrovandi and his contemporaries, it was all *legenda*—things to read' (Foucault, 2005, 44).[7] In the case of New Spain specifically, we know that Juan de la Fuente who would be the University of Mexico's first professor of medicine, held in his personal library works by Sebastian Brandt, Ovid, Terence, Antonio de Nebrija, Cicero and Erasmus; indeed, upon his death, one of the books in his personal library could not be located because Francisco Cervantes de Salazar, the philosopher, translator and author of the canonical *Crónica de la Nueva España* [Chronicle of New Spain] (1575), had borrowed it from his friend and had not returned it.[8] The arenas of medicine, academic enquiry, governance and high culture were intimately connected at this early stage in the development of New Spain's civic apparatus. The choice of medical texts as a point of departure is not arbitrary but rather brings into sharper focus the history of science in relation to literary activity. 'Science' in the early modern period and the Enlightenment, as Mary Baine Campbell recalls, 'was mostly still being written by writers, only some of them writing as scientists', a term that would not be used with the sense it is given today until

7 Foucault is referring to Georges-Louis Leclerc, Comte de Buffon, the eighteenth-century French naturalist who is considered a key figure in the history of biological sciences. Buffon would be one of the leading voices that argued for the innate inferiority of *criollos* to Europeans, an idea he advanced in his *Histoire naturelle* (1749). On the subject of how his ideas were challenged by intellectuals in the Americas, see Deans-Smith (2005).

8 For studies on what is known about the books Fuente brought with him to Mexico, as well as the titles he later declared before the Inquisition during the purge of 1571–72, see Martínez Hernández (2014, 207–11), as well as Viesca-Treviño and Aceves-Pastrana (2011, 455).

a later period (1999, 25).[9] To construe narrative elements as extra-scientific excess in medical books, or as separate from the epistemological production of scientific knowledge, speaks more to our present-day frameworks than to those of the early modern writer. And if the vehicle with which to arrive at scientific certainties at the time was prose, are not the considerations common to linguistic and literary texts also relevant to that process? What kind of science was is possible to make with linguistic tools and materials that also spoke of European expectations and biases?

During the sixteenth and early seventeenth centuries the medical literature of Europe would help to raise what were then a set of culturally and historically embedded epistemological practices from a comparatively small part of the world in a global scale to a platform where they demanded universal status. Scientific endeavour, and the written texts on which it relied for the dissemination of its findings, became part of a larger claim of civilisational superiority in the context of overseas expansion and growth. So strong did this model become by the end of the so-called Scientific Revolution that even despite wave after wave of superseded data, with the tried and true solutions of one generation becoming the toxic remedies or the inexact measurements of the next, still the underlying structure employed to generate new information would not be called into question.[10] In its ontology, early modern science devised mechanisms

9 Although the term 'scientist' is often accepted as having been coined in English in the nineteenth century by Campbell and by other sources including the OED, purportedly inspired from the word 'artist' according to the latter, the use of 'científico' as an adjective linked to empiricism is documented in Spanish well before. The *Diccionario de autoridades* in 1729 not only used it as a noun to refer to 'a person with expertise in some, or in many sciences, from the Latin *Scientificus* meaning the same', but importantly for our discussion, opposed 'scientific demonstration' to 'narration and entertainment' in one of its examples. It is likely the word had had a broader meaning that acquired a narrower use over time as more specific vocabulary became necessary to describe the work of emerging disciplines. Whether the declination of 'scientist' in English in the nineteenth century would have been at all influenced by similar philological practices in romance languages has not been determined.

10 In the first line of the introduction to his book on the subject, Steven Shapin playfully concedes that '[t]here was no such thing as the Scientific Revolution, and this is a book about it' (1). The cheeky paradox about the phrase, which was not in regular use prior to 1939, signals to sceptical readers that he is aware of the label's problematic standing today: 'as our understanding of science in the seventeenth century has changed', he explains, 'historians have become increasingly uneasy with the very idea' and 'now reject even the notion that there was any single coherent cultural entity called "science" [during that period] to undergo revolutionary change' (Shapin, 2018, 2, 3). In my own analysis, I refer to the 'so-called Scientific revolution', deliberately placed in quotation marks, both as a way of agreeing with the view that deems it a dated framework, but also to not lose sight of the substantial limiting effects this notion has historically placed on our ability to apprehend science-making in places that became colonial settings, before and after the arrival of Europeans.

that anticipated and contained its failures, redefining them as recurring but at the same time non-representative outputs, the necessary by-products of a process operating as it should, its perceived efficiency unscathed. Non-western epistemological approaches would largely be either rejected and condemned, or disarmed and re-christened as local 'practices' or 'traditions', to wit, unscientific ways of generating knowledge. Meanwhile, Europe's own cultural gestures for coding experiential memory, closely guarded by its social elites, would be raised as the only possible unfettered and unbiased position before the world: empiricism would become a Western prerogative and a cornerstone of modernity.

The writers discussed over the pages that follow, of course, had no way of knowing this would happen. Arias de Benavides, López de Hinojosos, Farfán and Cárdenas, were all born in the vicinity of major Spanish cities and came to the New World not as explorers but to join communities that were already in the making. In many ways, their texts were meant to be an integral part of the advancement of early modern European science in its march toward empiricism. But they will stumble in an encounter with coloniality, which sent them off on a different course. 'Coloniality', as Walter Mignolo explains expanding on Aníbal Quijano's definition, can be said to be 'the hidden logic of modernity', Renaissance Europe's attempt to disqualify 'all possible loci of enunciation [other than its own] from religious to economic, from legal to political, from ethical to erotic' as it expanded beyond its physical borders in projects of competing territorial expansion; there would be a 'right religion' and 'right ways of learning' (2003, 442). Initially torchbearers in that process, over the course of the second half of the sixteenth century, the Spaniards composing medical texts overseas begin to intuit that they would not be made full partners in the end. The increasing commodification and classification of American *materia medica* from afar would go on, with or without their assistance. Instead of an advantage, they found that their embeddedness in New World societies was perceived as eroding rather than enhancing the reach of their findings by European counterparts; other voices were glad to speak for them. The response to their newfound marginality would play out in the context of science, either by contesting the epistemological basis of claims made by authors who did not have their dual life experience (Benavides, Cárdenas) or, to a lesser degree, by turning away from a world stage altogether and redirecting attention to the local, foregoing the expectation that their books would reach a reader outside their communities (Hinojosos, and especially Farfán). Because this exercise was rehearsed in print, the traces of that performance in the texts complicate current models that situate the power divide in colonial structures between *peninsulares* and *criollos*, that is, Spaniards born in Spain, and colonial subjects claiming direct Spanish ascendancy, often accompanied by claims of racial 'purity'. Then as now, the politics of identity and allegiance to place and community for subjects in transit was considerably less straightforward.

Despite the methodological challenges of arriving at a definition that accounts for its complexity in the context of the early modern world, race remains a key consideration in many discussions about how difference between human beings was understood and policed in colonial Latin America. After all, as Irene Silverblatt notes, 'Iberian colonialism' played a pivotal role in making 'race-thinking' a 'way of life', for it was Spain and Portugal who undertook 'the first waves of colonialism [that] inaugurated the global, racialised categories of humanity with which we are only too familiar today' (2009, xi, x). But as Daniel Nemser has recently argued, while the idea of race in a place like sixteenth-century Mexico is linked to period understandings on ethnicity, it should not be thought of 'as an attribute or property of a particular body but as an effect of the material practices of power' in which 'the process of racialization' equated to 'the production of group-differentiated vulnerability' (2017, 9, 12). 'There was no Indian', Nemser reminds us, when Europeans first arrived (2017, 27); no single, overarching category that accounted for the intricate ways in which the various communities of the Americas understood themselves or their relationships to one another. The term would only become 'a meaningful category of identity' by fashioning a 'homogeneous population' bound by the physical and social constraints placed upon it 'out of a heterogeneous mosaic of indigenous forms of humanity' (2017, 27). His point is well taken, among other reasons because it recognises the rise of colonial-era racial categories first and foremost as process, and as dynamic. The evolution of the region's racial frameworks would come to draw on both essentialist and constructionist arguments, reifying practices of exclusion even as it remained susceptible to changing contextual factors (Twinam, 2015, 42). 'Spanish America', Ann Twinam explains, 'was universalist and racist in its assignation of blackness as an inferior category justifying discrimination', but 'was constructionist in that it recognised variable statuses between white and black and brown and Spanish and African and Native and permitted movement among categories' (2015, 42–43).[11] The colonial era saw the progressive consolidation of modes of categorisation that relied on what were initially, in the late fifteenth and sixteenth centuries, unstable and arbitrary labels, not all of which would ultimately become 'meaningful', in Nemser's sense, or would even survive into later periods.

New analytical approaches grounded more firmly in the disciplines of history and political science are helpful in that they provide panoramic assessments on how the process of racialisation unfolded in the region, but they can remain somewhat on the fence when it comes to locating agency; the who-did-the-unfolding, as it were. In our attempts to distance ourselves from patriarchal narratives of the past overly concerned with the actions of a handful of figures endowed with protagonist status, it can seem as if we are then relegating human agency and decision-making to the background,

11 Twinam, expanding on Ann Laura Stoler's definition of essentialist and constructionist approaches to race, prefers to use 'socioracial' rather than 'racial' status to underscore the tension between 'changeable variables' and the 'hierarchy [that] remained' (2015, 43).

having them appear as handmaidens to larger, unseen historical forces. This refocusing can hinder attempts at mapping and gauging the range of actions (and reactions), individual and collective, that had an impact in giving greater credence to certain period views on race over others. Along with a consideration of foundational events or prescriptive measures, such as proclamations and edicts made by the Catholic Church and the Crown, one can ask what choices at the level of quotidian responses to ongoing developments in New Spain either fuelled, witnessed or resisted the cyphering of racial categories so as to enable them to take shape in the way they did and not along different lines. Does new information come to light if we pay greater attention to what could be termed catalyst, or cul-de-sac classification attempts, that is, modes of describing difference and group identity that were proposed at the time, and that may have resonated with readers in conversations relevant to race, but that were ultimately displaced within colonial discourse? The surgical and medical literature of New Spain provides an unexpectedly useful platform from which to begin answering some of those questions.

In the sixteenth century, there was not a consensus on the use of racial lexicon, or more precisely, on lexicon that did the work of race, extending into considerations about *calidad*.[12] The terminology created by Europeans to demarcate group identities along ethnic and racial lines in the Americas sometimes turned to neologisms, many of them phonetic renderings in Spanish of Indigenous voices (*caribe*, *taíno*), but it also recycled existing words that called to mind 'exotic' geographic settings (*indios*, *negros guineos*), or that were used to refer to non-humans in arenas like plant cultivation and horse breeding (*mestizo*, *mulato*).[13] The medical books of early colonial Mexico reflect these fluctuations and imprecisions. Sometimes it is clear that the author is referring to an 'español' or an 'indio', but often it is not; at times, the race of a body under examination is of the essence to illustrate the writer's point, but in other moments it does not come across as a matter of consequence. The socio-historical circumstances in which these works were produced and circulated, namely New Spain as it was in the late sixteenth

12 María Elena Martínez explains that although it became more popular in later periods 'the concept of calidad was already used in the sixteenth century'; it would come to 'refe[r] to a number of factors, including economic status, occupation, purity of blood, and birthplace' (2008, 356). For an analysis of the appropriateness of using race to describe processes of differentiation in early colonial Latin America, see María Eugenia Chaves, whose work historicises scholarly debate on the issue up to the time of the output's publication (2012, 39–58).

13 On the use of terms like *taino* and *caribe* as ethnic markers, and the rejection by Kalinago peoples of the latter, see Stone (2018, 118–47). Ruth Hill's work has shown how some terminology used in the sixteenth century to describe human generation and racial mixing in parts of Spain and later in the Americas can be traced to *libros de albeitería* (veterinary books on horse breeding) and to botanical contexts. See Hill (2015, 45–64).

century, make it impossible for people who other period materials described as *mestizos*, *mulatos* and *criollos*—all terms already in circulation—, to have been hidden from view, and yet, surgical and medical authors only conjure up these categories obliquely, if at all. What does their textual absence in light of New Spain's demographic reality at that point in time reveal about local medical discourse and the readers whom it spoke to?

The term *mestizo*, which as Ruth Hill notes 'appears repeatedly in Gabriel Alonso de Herrera's 1513 *Agricultura*' (2015, 49) pertaining to botanical matters, was used in print to describe the offspring of Europeans and Indigenous people instead at least as far back as the first version of Fernández de Oviedo's *Historia general y natural de las Indias*, published in 1535 with a shorter title.[14] Oviedo wrote about *mestizos* not as a main point of interest but in passing, in a section focused on the Indigenous people of Hispaniola whom he claimed were of inferior character, prone to lying and lacking steadfastness. *Mestizos*, he contended, made this judgment irrefutable, illustrating how negative traits carried over into the next generation even in cases of partial European ancestry: 'And that what I have stated about the said Indians should be believed is proven by the *mestizos*, the children of Christian men and Indian women, because it is only with immense effort that they can be properly raised, and are capable of rejecting vices and wicked inclinations.'[15] *Mulato*, which Sebastián Covarrubias defined for readers of the following century in his *Tesoro de la lengua castellana o española* (1611) as the progeny of 'a Black woman and a white man, or the opposite, and being an extraordinary mixture it was compared to the nature of the mule', is a term thought to have circulated in Iberia early on in the sixteenth century.[16] It is present in Portuguese and Italian materials dating to the 1520s, and as Esperança Cardeira has found, evidence suggests that it went 'from Spanish or from Portuguese to Italian (*mulatto*) and then to French (*mulâtre*) and English (mulatto)' (2016, 81).[17] Both *mestizo* and *mulato* were well-established terms

14 In addition to the first edition, which appeared in Alcala de Henares, Herrera's text was published many times in Spain over the course of the sixteenth century, with at least five additional known printings before 1535.

15 'Y que se deba creer lo que tengo dicho de los indios pruébase por los mestizos hijos de cristianos e indias, porque con gravísimo trabajo se crían y pueden apartar de vicios y malas inclinaciones' (1535, 37r). The term also appears with the sense of being the offspring of Spaniards and Indigenous parents in Juan de la Cruz's *Doctrina christiana* printed in Mexico in 1571. However, as Hill observes, there is evidence in sixteenth-century and early seventeenth-century European sources of 'mestizo' also being used to refer to dogs, plants as well as to 'the offspring of a Moor and a White' (2015, 49).

16 'hijo de negra y hombre blanco, o al revés: y por ser mezcla extraordinaria la compararon a la naturaleza del mulo' (1998, 819).

17 Among the examples of early use Cardeira finds are Gil Vicente's *Tragicomédia de Dom Duardos* (c.1521–24), spoken by a Spanish character in the play, and a translation into Italian of a Portuguese source done by Ramusio in 1525 (81). Like *mestizo*, *mulato* also retained pejorative associations to zoological contexts. On the case of

in New Spain by the mid 1550s, used in materials such as cabildo documents without needing to be explained, their presence also decried by Indigenous elites who, as Robert C. Schwaller notes, felt 'dismayed by their impact on the social, economic and cultural order' (2016, 4).[18] *Criollo* was first used by the Portuguese to refer to enslaved Afro-Brazilians, and Ralph Bauer and José Antonio Mazzotti trace its presence in written sources with the sense of non-Black Europeans born in the New World to 'letters written during the 1560s by Spanish officials from New Spain' (2009, 4), materials which tended to mark them in this way to espouse negative views.[19]

Sidelining medical texts from New Spain because they do not consistently turn to these labels, or because they do not readily perform the distinguishing, classificatory gestures that became commonplace when it comes to race during the colonial era, misses the mark on why they are relevant to our understanding of the process of racialisation in Latin America. 'Other means of stereotyping, marginalizing or excluding the "other"', as Tamar Herzog observes, 'existed alongside, added to, and at times replaced, a discourse on race and it is only by integrating them into our analysis that we can come to understand fully the ways by which early modern individuals understood both similarities and differences' (2012, 153). In this vein, a literary analysis of the period's medical prose, including of its phrasing and lexical choices, brings us back to Nemser's idea of sixteenth-century New Spain as a 'heterogeneous [human] mosaic'—here referring to Indigenous peoples and also to the wider range of colonial subjects who occupied different positions along a spectrum of privilege and vulnerability. Combining the tools of literary studies and cultural studies brings into focus the role these books played in shaping colonial imaginaries and subjectivities, and the significance of whether or not local science chose to advance racialised models of human anatomy and physiology when and if it did.

It is worth noting that the disempowering racialisation of cultural 'others' of African and Indigenous ancestry that became a defining feature of European modes of colonisation in overseas territories did not preclude consonant, synchronous efforts within Iberia's own evolving socio-political landscape, reflecting its ongoing anxieties over cultural and ethnic diversity in emerging projects of national consolidation. These anxieties predated

mulato specifically and its links to medieval notions about degeneracy in the context of dogs and horse-breeding, see Beusterien (2016, 114–15).

18 For an in-depth study examining the socio-racial and political dimensions of these two categories helpfully focused on sixteenth-century New Spain, see Schwaller (2015).

19 According to Stephanie Merrim, 'the word *criollo*, which formerly referred to Afro-Brazilian slaves, first assumed the meaning of "American-born Spaniard" in a letter of 1567 [addressed to the Council of the Indies] branding creoles as troublemakers' (2010, 16). It is, therefore, reasonable to assume the term may have been used orally to convey a similar meaning before being set down in manuscript and print sources.

the contact with the Americas, and in Europe, they could be amplified or assuaged by events taking place in colonial peripheries as well. Going back to medieval times, as Herzog notes, 'one of the most powerful means of making distinctions in early modern Spain and Spanish America was the conceptual divide between community members (called *vecinos* when referring to the local community, *naturales* when referring to the various Iberian kingdoms) and foreigners' (2012, 153). Debates surrounding these distinctions, she adds,

> although focused on social and political membership … are important to the study of 'race' as an analytical category because they were employed not only to measure the degree of belonging to a political community but also as a generic discourse against any group whose members, because of their cultural, social or ethnic belonging could be considered external to the Spanish community. (2012, 155–56)

Identity groups understood as such, were placed along hierarchical axes, and their distance from more powerful sectors of Iberian society was differentially increased or minimised depending on context. Regional variations mattered too, for example, raising the status of some Spaniards above others depending on where in Spain they were from. Conversely, invoking a sense of Spanishness that did not dwell on regional or social differences could help to shift negative attention toward groups construed as alien because of their link to places physically outside Spain and Portugal, thus bolstering a sense of commonality between people native to the Peninsula. Sent back to Spain in chains in 1500, Columbus himself would be forced to reckon with the fact that, despite being a fellow Christian whose children lived at the Spanish court, and not one of the 'indios' he had so named, he was still 'un pobre extranjero' [a poor foreigner]—in the eyes of the Spanish monarchs he chided for their ingratitude, and to the Spanish settlers of Hispaniola who had risen up against him, demanding his arrest (1993, 109). It was no accident that sixty years on, Nicolás Monardes (discussed in chapters 1 and 4), a key figure in the history of early modern Hispanic science, pointedly began his influential *Historia medicinal* [Medicinal history] (1565) by reminding readers of their incalculable debt to 'Columbus, the Genoese'. Monardes, the Sevillian son of a Genoese bookseller, and a man born and raised in the city that then housed the largest Genoese settlement outside of that republic, implied with this gesture that his countrymen perhaps ought to adopt a similarly appreciative stance toward his own service of writing a book that unveiled the Americas' splendid medicinal wealth, a treasure that surpassed all its other riches in his view, not for his own personal gain but for that of Spain.[20]

20 Monardes (1565, fol. 1r). The Genoese had their own quarter within the city, with its own shops, public baths and church. It also enjoyed some autonomy when it came to deciding internal judicial matters. For a fuller discussion of Monardes and the Genoese community in Seville at the time, see Pérez Marín (2006, 36, 49–51).

If we accept Rolena Adorno's argument on the centrality of text and of narrative as a genre in the origins of Latin American literary culture, a closer look at the kinds of dialogue medical books sustained with the literature and historiography of the period can add a new dimension to our understanding of the evolution of Latin American letters. Referring both to the chronicles of military leaders like Hernán Cortés and the work of Indigenous historians such as Felipe Guaman Poma de Ayala, Adorno contends that their works 'do not describe events; they *are* events', with 'colonial writing [being] a social practice, rather than merely a reflection of it' (2007, 4). Under that analytical framework, Church edicts, conversion manuals and medical texts can also be thought of as events; just not big events; rather everyday events that became embedded in the routines and daily interactions of New Spain's inhabitants. When brought into the fold of literary and cultural studies, medical writers may follow less grandiose itineraries than the ones charted by the major historical figures of the canon but theirs can be equally compelling. The reward of not neglecting this body of work is that it reveals the lived experience of colonial subjects in its diversity, granting this sector the attention it is denied elsewhere. Printed books on medicine are but one site of colonial enunciation among many others and do not represent a shared or unified New World mentality. The overwhelming number of voices that spoke in early modern Latin America were not captured by the printed page nor is it wise to try to reduce their plurality. But literary analysis, when used to study materials as preoccupied with the needs of local communities as were surgical and medical texts, can help us hear beyond the audible spectrum, through passages that are often just as interested in conveying information on anatomical structures as they are in telling us about the people whose bodies they belonged to.

The sections in *Marvels of Medicine* offer four main entry points into New World medical literature of the second half of the sixteenth century, organised along a broad chronological arc. Chapter 1, 'The surgeon's secrets: the medical travel narrative of Pedro Arias de Benavides', explores the *Secretos de Chirurgia* [Secrets of Surgery] (1567), a text written by a Spanish surgeon who travelled throughout the Caribbean, Mexico and Central America in the mid-sixteenth century. Part surgical manual, part medieval book of secrets, part voyage diary, the *Secretos* weaves together medical and anatomical information alongside extended personal accounts of the author's experiences in the Americas. Giving rise to a hybrid form that shares in the poetics of earlier encounter-period literature, with its emphasis on discovery and revelation, the *Secretos* is at the same time a work of science. My analysis reveals the discursive slippage in Benavides's language, where the notion of the 'secret' becomes an errant topic that metaphorically codes the inner body as a new *terra incognita* to be known, tamed and conquered. Like Cabeza de Vaca and Díaz del Castillo, Benavides placed himself at the centre of his tale and offered lively vignettes on the events he witnessed and the people he met. But as a relatively minor player in the context of Iberian territorial expansion, the voices that come through in his text are not those of conquistadors or of major political figures but of the everyday men and women who enter the page as patients, associates and neighbours, thus capturing points of view seldom given sustained consideration in other kinds of colonial-era historiography. My reading also highlights Benavides's innovative use of medical illustrations, namely shapes for incisions and instrument designs, several of which are printed life-size and transform the text into a surgical instrument in and of itself. By comparing marginalia present in the surviving copies of the *Secretos*, I offer a roadmap into the range of chronicled and also possible period responses to the text on the part of its early modern readers. Printed in Spain, but sold in Europe as well as in the Americas, the text's frequent humorous anecdotes betray a growing unease at the marginal status assigned to members of overseas communities by European authorities. Benavides's writing anticipates strategies of resistance to colonial rule that would eventually come to characterise *criollo* discourse. As a precursor to the satirical writings of a figure like Juan del Valle y Caviedes, and as the work of a European who continued to identify with a New World community even after returning to the continent, the *Secretos* calls into question the extent to which the *peninsular/criollo* divide is a useful distinction when examining texts written in colonial Mexico during its foundational period, before the seventeenth century.

Chapter 2, 'Irreconcilable differences? Anatomy, physiology and the New World body', seeks to outline the limits of a normative notion of the body in colonial medical discourse during the last third of the sixteenth century. It centres on a close reading of two important writers in this context: Alonso López de Hinojosos and Juan de Cárdenas. Despite lacking a university education and working primarily as a nurse practitioner, with the *Svmma, y recopilacion de chirvgia* [Surgical compendium] (1578, 1595), Hinojosos became the author of the first medical book printed in Spanish in the Americas. Cárdenas, on the other hand, was trained in medicine at the University of Mexico, part of its first cohort of graduates and, unlike Hinojosos's *Svmma*, which was primarily an anatomical and surgical manual, his own *Primera parte de los problemas y secretos marauillosos de las Indias* [First part of the problems and marvellous secrets of the Indies] (1591) centred on questions of natural history and physiology. Both Hinojosos's and Cardenas's treatment of New World bodies had a different resonance in the context of late sixteenth-century Mexico compared to similar discussions then unfolding in Europe, where strong arguments were being made for radical differences between the physiology of Spaniards and those belonging to other 'nations' [*naciones*]. Although the fact that in the case of Indigenous populations this debate is most often associated with theology and natural law, or with events like the Valladolid Debate, medicine is yet another crucial site of enunciation in colonial discourse where the question of a common human nature was raised. American medical texts (sometimes unwittingly) became satellite testing grounds for emerging European ideas, not just on social cohesion, but also on racial difference. The juxtaposition of Old World notions of corporeality with New World medical observations were both metaphorical and literal, given the reliance on Nahua bodies at times as a source from which to mine anatomical information then enlisted in the care and for the benefit of non-Indigenous patients. Despite their shared context and concern with medicine, when the *Svmma* and the *Problemas y secretos*[21] are placed side by side, anatomy and physiology become locked in a colonial paradox. Anatomy would find accumulating evidence of a repeating body template whose structures and behaviours seemed largely unaffected by a subject's ethnic background. But physiology, on the other hand, began to advance ideas on the purportedly measurable and differential potential of racialised bodies, seen as entities that performed differently in arenas like resistance before disease or predisposition toward intellectual achievement. At the heart of this oppositional tension lay the reality of a growing *mestizo* population, whose widespread but incomplete exclusion from consideration in medical literature speaks to the anxiety over its classification and sets the limits on how bodies in colonial society could be made intelligible.

Chapter 3, 'Weakening the sex: the medicalisation of female gender identity in New Spain', addresses the link between colonial ideas on proper femininity and period understandings of gendered physiology. Similar to their European counterparts in that they deemed women to have a weaker constitution compared to men, medical authors in New Spain, however, began linking their arguments on the female body to American environments specifically. Unlike the case of Spanish male subjects, who were able to draw some benefits from the cold and wet nature of the region that tempered their hot and dry humours, women's bodies were instead debilitated when subjected to the same conditions. Descriptions of physiological processes thus become part of arguments in favour of stricter controls on women's diets and behaviour in the New World under the guise of ensuring their good health. The rising numbers of European women in early colonial Mexico are reflected in the fact that the two locally printed medical books that go into second editions in the sixteenth century—Hinojosos's *Svmma* (1578, 1592) and Agustín Farfán's *Tractado breve de anothomia y chirvgia* [Brief treatise on anatomy and surgery] (1579, 1592)—both revise and abridge their first versions in order to make way for new sections focused solely on the treatment of women and children. My analysis traces notions on gender, particularly in the case of 'exceptional' gestational processes resulting in manly women [*mujeres hombrunas*] and effeminate men [*hombres amarionados*] to sources including Damián Carbón's *Libro del arte delas Comadres, o madrinas* [Book of the art of midwives] (1541), showing how authors in the New World were bringing together under a colonial prism medical traditions that in Europe had taken divergent paths.

21 Cárdenas planned to write a second part to the text but it was never published. The text is commonly known today as the *Problemas y secretos maravillosos de las Indias* without the 'Primera parte'.

Paradoxically, in the case of Farfán's work, the interest in female medical problems and their bodily shortcomings opened a textual space for women's voices, given the author's tendency to recount exchanges with patients when providing supporting evidence about treatments. Farfán's remarks on the difficulties of tending to female patients, whose responses he portrayed as ranging from cooperative to highly sceptical of his advice, and whose all-too frequent unhealthy habits were cited as a common source of self-inflicted illness, bear witness to their high level of agency in matters relating to health. Farfán's concern with providing information that his readers would find useful leads him to address issues from perspectives not usually adopted by Hinojosos or other period sources, discussing matters like women's personal comfort, beauty routines, or the benefits of an active sex life independent of procreation aims. The intimate and self-reflexive nature of his text, and the compassion with which he considers issues of pain management, invite male practitioners and readers to consider a female embodied experience, anticipating narrative features associated with later forms of literature.

Chapter 4, 'Contested medical knowledge and regional self-fashioning', returns to Cárdenas's *Problemas y secretos* in the context of the negative critiques he offered of two contemporaries who had written about New World medicine without leaving Spain: Nicolás Monardes in Seville and Oliva Sabuco de Nantes Barrera in Alcaraz. Monardes's *Historia medicinal* [Medicinal history] (1565) was one of the most widely read medical texts on *materia medica* in Europe during the time, enjoying 25 printings in multiple languages in the sixteenth century alone, and becoming a standard source of reference in natural histories and medical books well into the seventeenth century. Sabuco, for her part, claimed an extra-academic educational and professional training, as the daughter of a pharmacist and just 25 years old at the time of the publication of the *Nveva filosofia de la naturaleza del hombre* [New philosophy on human nature] (1578). While Sabuco's authorship has been contested since the early twentieth century (still a matter of intense debate among early modern Hispanists, with some claiming the text was penned by her father rather than by her), my analysis sets aside that controversy to focus instead on the implications of Cárdenas's critique, for he wrote about the text believing it to be the work of a woman. Indeed, independently of its subject matter, the intertextual relationship with the *Nveva filosofia* makes the *Problemas y secretos* one of the earliest known sources in American writing to ever discuss in print the merits of a female author's ideas about any topic.

Cárdenas found fault with both the *Historia medicinal* and the *Nveva filosofia*, attacking Monardes's claims on the usefulness of bezoars, and Sabuco's model for the process of digestion. In both cases, his approach was to identify flaws in the cause and effect reasoning being espoused in the source and to provide examples that arrived at a different result. But Cárdenas's medical challenge, articulated on scientific principle, belied a growing unease regarding the marginal status conferred to locally published scholarly efforts in the larger global stage of scientific enquiry.

Monardes was keenly interested not just in bezoars but in New World bezoars especially; Sabuco's ideas on digestion rested on her observations of the quick effects of ingesting coca leaves from Peru, proof according to her that there had to be a structure connecting the mouth and the brain in addition to the stomach. For Cárdenas, experiments with specimens imported into European gardens and wonder cabinets were no substitute for the *in situ* observations New World medical practitioners stood to contribute. By adopting an oppositional model of refutation that anchored itself on a geographically and culturally determined group identity, one that went beyond a *peninsular/criollo* divide, Cárdenas's writing simultaneously anticipated and departed from the defensive discursive strategies of later thinkers in Spanish America who would go on to challenge the unequal distribution of power in colonial hierarchies.

To end the book, I include an epilogue reflecting on the cross-fertilisation between science and medicine on the one hand, and literature and art on the other in the consolidation of New World *criollo* identity and discourse, beyond the sixteenth century. It invites readers to consider two towering figures in the cultural history of colonial Latin America, writer Inca Garcilaso de la Vega and painter Miguel Cabrera, discussing each one's connection to earlier texts on anatomy and physiology. This final section argues for redefining the medical texts studied in *Marvels of Medicine* as early matrixes of colonial rhetoric, scientific as well as literary objects that charted a course for future colonial subjects' sense of identity in relation to the larger context of global knowledge production.

CHAPTER 1

The surgeon's secrets

The medical travel narrative of Pedro Arias de Benavides

Although expensive and relatively hard to come by depending on where you lived, dragon's blood was not exactly new in the context of sixteenth-century Spain. Known and prized in ancient times for giving a rich, deep red tint to artists' pigments, and mentioned by sources dating as far back as Dioscorides in the first century AD all the way to Bernardo de Gordonio in the fourteenth century, it was well known enough for renowned humanist physician Andrés Laguna to clarify in 1555 that the 'vulgar dragon's blood' then being sold in some medicine shops was not to be confused with the ingredient that had been described by Pliny the Elder, which the Roman author had claimed needed to be sourced from actual dragons. It was instead, Laguna affirmed, the same tree resin recorded by Dioscorides, 'that fiery-coloured liqueur very familiar to painters, which is commonly called dragon's blood'.[1] Because of its intense hue, 'some had once been persuaded' it came from these mythical creatures, but this superseded idea was relevant only to understanding its name, which endured 'even in our times'.[2] The expanding early modern medicine cabinet had brought dragon's blood onto the page once again, and the 'discovery' by Europeans of resins thought to be that substance, first in the Canary Islands and then in the Americas, had renewed discussion. One salient voice on the matter would be that of Nicolás Monardes[3] who over a decade after Laguna's remarks, and notwithstanding the more prosaic position of his celebrated colleague on the matter (Laguna was, after all, a physician to a pope and to kings), in his second and expanded 1571 edition of the *Historia medicinal*

1 Laguna writes: 'el verdadero cinabrio de los antiguos no es otra cosa, sino aquel encendido licor, y a los pintores muy familiar, que vulgarmente se dice sangre de drago' (1555, 540).

2 According to Laguna, '[t]iene aqueste un color muy penetrante, y sanguíneo, de do se persuadieron algunos, que fuese sangre de drago: el cual nombre le dura hasta estos tiempos' (1555, 540).

3 For recent discussions on Monardes's treatment of dragon's blood and on the disambiguation on the various substances that were given that name, see Bauer, 'The Blood of the Dragon' (2014, 67–88), and chapter 9 of *The Alchemy of Conquest* (2019).

[Medicinal history] (1565) reported seeing a tiny dragon inside a fruit that had been picked from a dragon's blood tree.[4] It had been brought to Monardes in Seville from Terra Firme by the Bishop of Cartagena who had shared it with him on account of the holy man being 'learned and curious' and, as he adds somewhat immodestly, 'a fan of the book we had written'.[5] The description in the second edition of the *Historia* brims with suspense: 'I wanted to see it, so we opened one leaf, which is where the seed lies, and once opened there appeared a dragon made with such artifice that it seemed alive, its neck long, the mouth open, thorny hackles raised, with spikes, the tail long and standing on its feet.'[6] This singular experience leads Monardes to forcefully reject, even mock, other possible explanations for the naming of the tree and its resin such as the one that had been offered by Laguna, etymological or otherwise, claiming the real reason was instead the amazing hidden find. The novelty of his self-proclaimed breakthrough is further highlighted for readers with a full folio-sized illustration depicting the fruit whole and then sliced in half, with the dragon resting atop the bottom slice.[7] The compositional layout of the image multiplies what in the prose is just one physical specimen into three iterating visual objects, thus extending the reach of his underlying claim, namely, the implication that miniature, hidden dragons were a defining feature of the tree species as a whole. Pedro Arias de Benavides, like Laguna, had no time for such nonsense. In his *Secretos de Chirurgia* [Secrets of Surgery] (1567), this contemporary of Monardes had already warned readers about what he saw as a rising trend among fellow authors writing on American nature who seemed to him to be moved more by a desire for personal profit and self-aggrandisement than by the pursuit of facts. 'This is a tree', explained Benavides, 'that all or most authors have written on, but not about its shape and manner; I have seen it, so I will tell the truth.'[8]

4 Laguna was a figure of excellent standing at the time, physician to Pope Julius III at the time and later to both Charles V and Philip II. His translation of Dioscorides enjoyed wide circulation. The 1555 *editio princeps* was published in Antwerp; four others followed, printed in Salamanca in 1563, 1566, 1570 and 1586 (Miguel Alonso, 2020).

5 '[E]l Obispo de Cartagena varón religiosísimo, y docto, y muy curioso en estas cosas el cual me buscó luego en llegando [a Sevilla], porque estaba aficionado al libro que hicimos, desta materia herbaria' (1571, fol. 91r).

6 '[Y]o lo quise ver, y abrimos una hoja do está la simiente, y abierta la hoja apareció un dragón hecho con tanto artificio, que parecía vivo, el cuello largo, la boca abierta, el cerro en erizado, con espinas, la cola larga, y puesto en sus pies' (1571, fol. 91v).

7 This image has enjoyed a relatively high level of visibility in recent years compared to other period *materia medica* illustrations, appearing not just in studies about Monardes but associated also to scholarly projects on early modern Iberian medicine or the history of scientific illustration more broadly. See, for example, Slater et al., *Medical Cultures* (2014) and Cabezas et al., *Dibujo científico* (2016).

8 'Este es un árbol que todos los autores o los más, escriben de él, y no la forma y manera de él. [Y]o le he visto, y diré la verdad de él' (1567, fol. 53v).

In some ways, Benavides is playing both sides. As in the case of other natural products and medicines featured in the *Secretos*, he sought to capitalise on the allure dragon's blood would have held for his contemporaries, an interest fuelled by the language of wonder and amazement increasingly associated with spaces of exploration and European expansion. But once they arrive at the text, he proceeds to debunk the air of mystique that led them there in the first place. Benavides draws audiences in with the promise of information on the latest surgical techniques, remedies for serious and high-sounding diseases of the day, and news on exotic medicines from the Indies being dangled before readers by the likes of Monardes. Yet the reward of his own project, as he saw it, lay in stripping New World medicine of myth and mystery to unveil its practical but ultimately real value. In the case of dragon's blood, first he dispels embellished notions about the tree's appearance, noting in detail the colour and texture of its bark, and he then describes how local people used the resin for dental hygiene, which gave them strong teeth and sweet breath.[9] As will be the case throughout the book when discussing plants and insects, Benavides's observations go beyond health applications into contextual matters, commenting on the usefulness of the tree's wood for fashioning war shields and speculating as to what would be the ideal weather conditions for it to thrive. He emphasises that he has personally seen dragon's blood harvested in El Hierro (one of the islands in the Canaries archipelago), and laments that so much misinformation circulated about its provenance. Underscoring autobiographical experience, the section ends with a disparaging allusion to those who write 'por relación', that is, from what they have been told instead of what they have witnessed, authors who unlike him were not first-hand observers. 'I know of some', quips Benavides, 'principally the physicians of Seville, who on account of *relaciones* and letters have written some things; I will concern myself here to write only of what I have seen, and many times experienced.'[10] If we take into consideration that the first edition of Monardes's best-selling *Historia medicinal* had been published in 1565, and that the *Secretos* appeared but two years later, it is likely that at least one of the targets of his pointed remark was none other than the celebrated Sevillian doctor who would go on to write so colourfully about dragon's blood, continuing to garner ever-increasing fame all over Europe for his foray into American *materia medica*, even if, as Benavides would stress, as no more than an armchair traveller.[11]

9 See Benavides (1567, fol. 54r).

10 'Yo sé de algunos, principalmente que los médicos de Sevilla, por relaciones y cartas han escrito algunas cosas yo no procuraré aquí sino decir lo que he visto, y las cosas que muchas veces he experimentado' (1567, fol. 54v).

11 For a discussion on how Monardes's *Historia medicinal* was read and critiqued by authors writing in Mexico in the late sixteenth century, see chapter 4. If true that Benavides may be alluding to Monardes in this line, José Luis Fresquet Febrer notes that he would have come across his colleague's work at an advanced stage in the writing process, or after having already completed the manuscript (1993, 68).

From our vantage point today looking at the history of Iberian science, it is tempting to place Monardes and Benavides on equal footing, that is on the side of early modern scholars who ascribed a positive value to American nature, and who insisted upon making personal observation a primary basis of epistemological authority, irrespective of whether new findings went against the grain of earlier sources. We would recall that theirs was not a position that could be taken for granted at this historical juncture given that in European scholarly circles the tide had not yet fully turned in favour of empiricism as a means for establishing universal truths, nor was 'experience' defined in the terms the so-called Scientific Revolution would insist upon later in the seventeenth century albeit, as I discuss in the introduction, with its own prejudices and socio-cultural limitations when engaging non-Western systems of thought.[12] By choosing to give sensorial observation a privileged status, one worthy of informing the daily practice and published findings of a physician, both authors departed from the established academic stance that regarded the natural products of the Americas with a degree of suspicion compared to those of the Far East that had longer documented uses in Western sources. However, as Benavides's own words lay bare, he and Monardes would have made uncomfortable bedfellows. He did not think very highly of physicians who managed to acquire limited samples for their private collections or botanical gardens and then claimed a thorough understanding of matters on that basis. Condescendingly, and perhaps with a tinge of envy, he reminds his readers that these authors 'are people reluctant to give up the good life and riches they have', and were either unwilling or incapable of engaging in the kind of travel and research that he had performed.[13] Being an eyewitness implied more than making contact with a given plant or animal part from the comfort and safety of one's own home, in Europe. Monardes may have presented his findings as first-hand experience, but for Benavides along with other authors who would voice the same concerns in Mexico and Peru over the next 50 years (as I discuss in chapter 4), that kind of engagement did not reach the epistemological standard that would have allowed it to be defined as experience proper.

12 Here I follow Antonio Barrera-Osorio's work on what he terms Spain's 'Early Scientific Revolution', a period in the sixteenth century which 'saw the consolidation of empirical scientific activities', but that still 'remained rooted in commercial and political interests without completely establishing its goals, rules, and epistemological conditions' (2006, 5, 10).

13 'Porque es gente que no quiere dejar la buena vida y riquezas que allá tienen' (1567, 54v–55r). In the same passage, he claims that, with the exception of a certain 'Robles' who returned to Salamanca from Peru, no other surgeon before him had traveled back to Spain from the Indies. There are, however, mentions of other European medical practitioners in earlier narratives, such as Diego Álvarez Chanca who accompanied Columbus on his second voyage and wrote about his experience, so it may be Benavides was unfamiliar with them.

As far as the *Secretos* was concerned, in order to know or to speak of new worlds, one had to have lived in them.

The *Secretos de Chirurgia, especial de las enfermedades de Morbo galico y Lamparones y Mirrarchia, y assi mismo la manera como se curan los Indios de llagas y heridas y otras pasiones en las Indias, muy util y provechoso para España y otros muchos secretos de chirurgia hasta agora no escriptos* [*Secrets of surgery: particularly on the French disease, and scrofula, and mirarchia, as well as the manner in which the Indians cure themselves of blisters and wounds and other afflictions in the Indies, very useful and valuable for Spain and other many secrets of surgery never before written*] presents itself in its lengthy title as an authoritative source on some of the more troublesome sicknesses of the day (see figure 1.1). 'Morbo gálico' [French disease] also referred to as 'bubas' in the text, was one of the names given to a spectrum of symptoms that (rightly or wrongly) would come to be associated with syphilis in later centuries.[14] 'Lamparones', today known as scrofula, were abscesses found around the neck caused by a disorder of the lymph nodes, and were called 'King's Evil' in early modern England given the belief that they could be cured by a monarch's touch. 'Mirrarchia' (atypically spelled by Benavides with a double 'r') referred to an inflammatory disease of the peritoneum.[15] In addition to these three headlining illnesses, the title twice alludes to the Indies, as a geographic location and by promising to share insights about Indigenous practices, not just products, a consideration that progressively recedes into the background as the colonial project gets under way.[16] By

14 In this chapter as well as in the rest of the book, I will avoid translating terms like 'morbo gálico' or 'bubas' into syphilis, both to mark the significance of linguistic choices in a given historical context, but also to allow for the possibility that period sources were describing more than a single pathogen, in light of what we know today about the symptoms and rates of transmission for that bacterial infection which do not map neatly onto early modern medical descriptions. There is not a consensus among present-day historians of medicine that mentions of 'morbo gálico', 'bubas' or even 'syphilis' refer to the disease known today by the latter label. Benavides does not address the apparent contradiction of using a French name for the illness, accepting Juan de Vigo's view of an American origin, and noting that it would go by various names after 'Columbus ... and those that came with him' had brought it back to Europe (fol. 11v). See chapter 2 for a fuller discussion of this topic.

15 'Mirarchia' is discussed in Jaume Roig's *Spill o Llibre de les dones* (1460) as well as in Fernando de Córdoba's *Suma de la flor de cirugia*, a manuscript source from the second half of the fifteenth century. It was one of many health problems that afflicted María of Castile, queen consort of Aragon. For information on Roig's treatment of the disease, see Solomon (1997, 82); for information on Córdoba's 'mirarchia' diagnosis, see Earenfight (2010, 191); for information on other period medical sources that used variants of the term 'miraque', see Pérez Pascual (1992, 759).

16 For a discussion of this issue in the context of late sixteenth-century Mexico and Agustín Farfán's medical writing, which resists this tendency, see Pérez Marín (2020, 103–16).

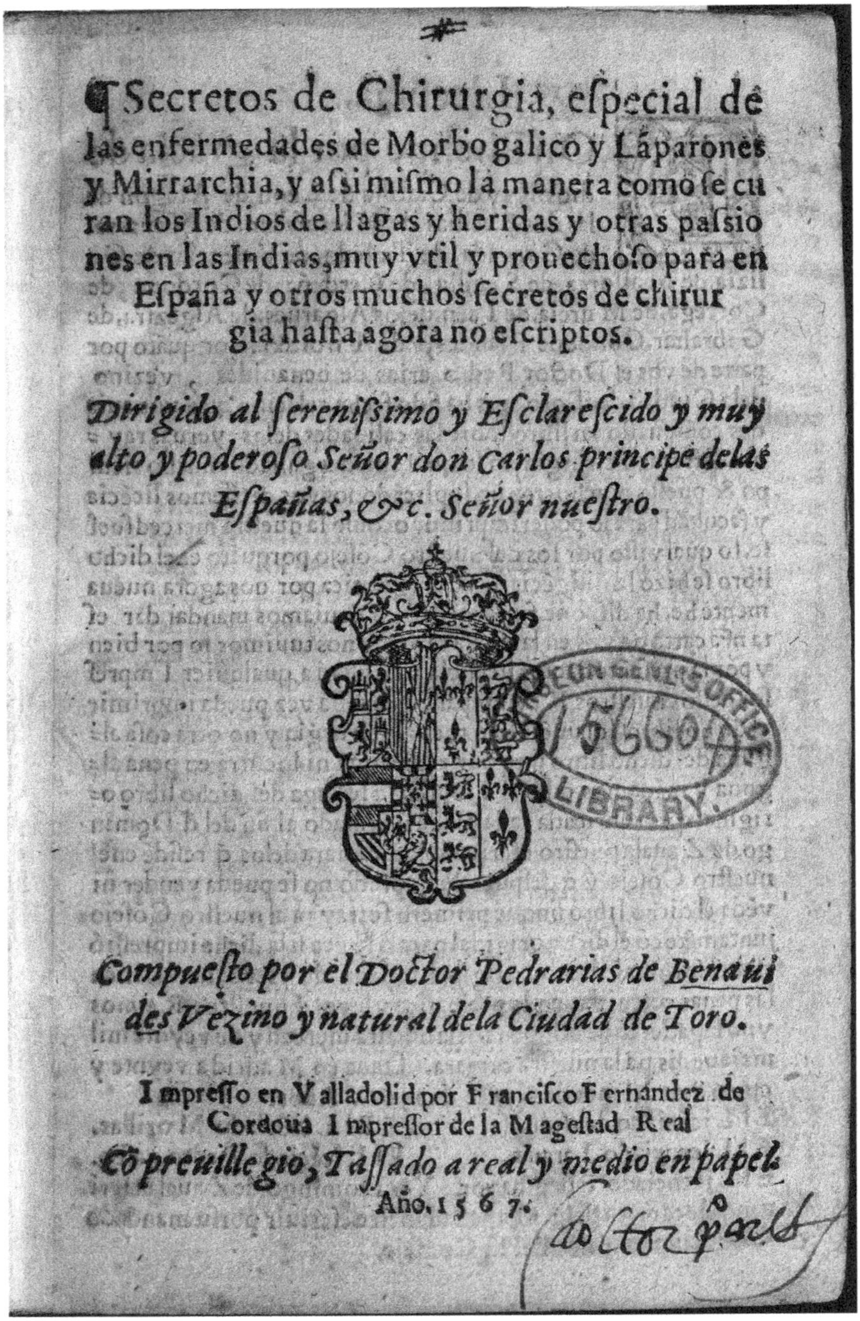

¶Secretos de Chirurgia, eſpecial dẽ
las enfermedades de Morbo galico y Laparones
y Mirrarchia, y aſsi miſmo la manera como ſe cu
ran los Indios de llagas y heridas y otras paſsio
nes en las Indias, muy vtil y prouechoſo para en
Eſpaña y otros muchos ſecretos de chirur
gia haſta agora no eſcriptos.

Dirigido al ſereniſsimo y Eſclareſcido y muy
alto y poderoſo Señor don Carlos principe delas
Eſpañas, &c. Señor nueſtro.

Compueſto por el Doctor Pedrarias de Benaui
des Vezino y natural dela Ciudad de Toro.

Impreſſo en Valladolid por Franciſco Fernandez de
Cordoua Impreſſor de la Mageſtad Real
Cõ preuillegio, Taſſado a real y medio en papel.
Año, 1567.

Figure 1.1. Title page of Pedro Arias de Benavides's *Secretos de Chirurgia* [Secrets of Surgery] (1567).
Courtesy of the US National Library of Medicine.

the middle of the sixteenth century, works on natural history or medicine relating to the Americas could lavish praise upon a medicinal product for its intrinsic properties at the same time that they denied any level of intellectual sophistication to the curative methods of Indigenous health practitioners. The success these societies had experienced with the medicinal simples around them was taken as fortunate yet incidental, not the result of a well-reasoned intellectual process. Instead, Benavides's book declared an interest not just in the substances found in the Indies but in how they were put to use by non-Europeans.[17] These divergences from the norm already hinted at in the title are a clue to some of the other features that make the *Secretos* an overlooked but extremely rich source for us today.

Few modern scholars have taken a serious interest in Benavides with the notable exception of José Luis Fresquet Febrer, who authored a monograph on the *Secretos* almost three decades ago and, more recently, Michael Solomon has offered a brief but enlivening close reading of the text's recommended treatment for penile fistulas.[18] The work usually receives little more than a passing mention in longer expositions about something else, and almost exclusively in the disciplinary context of the history of science and medicine rather than colonial Latin American literature or early modern studies.[19] One point often repeated is its purported status as the first comprehensive print medical source written by a European that highlighted Aztec medicine. But this watershed label is slippery and misleading, true only in a narrow sense as knowledge about curative Indigenous practices, some of them with possible Nahua origins, was already in circulation in earlier documents. There were also prior collaborative projects like the

17 The *Badianus Codex* (1552) is another source that departs from the norm in this regard. The codex centered on local flora and also paid considerable attention to Aztec mores and knowledge in its representation and organisation of the various remedies.

18 I am referring here to Fresquet Febrer's *La experiencia americana y la terapéutica en los Secretos de Chirurgia de Pedro Arias de Benavides* (1993), published as part of the Cuadernos Valencianos series, and Solomon (2010, 60–62, 94 and 96).

19 Prior to Fresquet Febrer's monograph, the *Secretos* had been discussed by Germán Somolinos d'Ardois in 1980 as part of his survey of Mexican medical texts (1980b, 196–97). In the nineteenth century, the book was mentioned by Joaquín García Icazbalceta (1954, 321), and by Anastacio Chinchilla (1841, 436–46), although both disclose not having handled a copy directly. Chinchilla's treatment is noteworthy because in his own survey of medical literature, focused on Spain rather than Latin America, he incorporates a chapter-by-chapter gloss of the *Secretos* that had been prepared by a colleague, identified as José Gutiérrez de la Vega. More recently, Benavides has been mentioned in passing by Barrera-Osorio (2006, 91, 122) and by Skaarup (2015, 203–04). It seems a curious coincidence that the section that most interests Solomon, dealing with the treatment of genital fistulas in a male patient, was deemed so noteworthy by Chinchilla that he transcribed it in full in his 1841 study, the only chapter of the text he opted to quote rather than summarise.

Badianus Codex,[20] which had approached the subject of local products and forms of treatment, albeit coding that information primarily in Latin rather than Castilian, and in manuscript form rather than in print. Lastly, as a work *about* the Americas but not published *in* the Americas, Francisco Bravo's *Opera medicinalia* (1570) and not the *Secretos* takes the title of the first printed American medical book proper. Scarcely mentioned in later sources, and lacking a modern edition, Benavides's text tends to be reduced to a colophon or a bibliographic curiosity. Yet the eccentric nature of the *Secretos* is one of its assets, holding information not found elsewhere and standing at the intersection of scientific investigation and voyage account, straying from what audiences of the time would have expected to find in a surgical treatise.

Neither the text nor the surviving historiography give up clues on whether Benavides's foray into the New World was associated with a particular commission or a financial venture, an unusual absence in the narrative economy of the *relación*, a genre so invested in highlighting successes and minimising failures before a patron back home. Benavides writes as if he were undecided about the kind of book he wants to assemble, with some sections that are more formulaic and other moments where readers are taken on a personal journey through the author's social encounters in a progression not always determined by medical considerations. The anomalous status of a medical book that is at once an extended travel narrative opens a window onto the daily lives of fledgling colonial communities in the New World, with an emphasis in New Spain. Time and again, he will share anecdotes about patients, about fellow surgeons who either supported or challenged his methods, about conversations with other members of his social circle, about people he met in passing, and about interactions with proportionally underrepresented figures in early modern literature and historiography, like *mestizos* and women of Indigenous and African descent. The level of access to the views and sensibilities of people living at the time that Benavides's text makes possible are not altogether different from those offered by works

20 The *Libellus de Medicinalibus Indorum Herbis*, known as the Badianus Codex, was dictated by Aztec medicine man Martín de la Cruz to Juan Badiano who translated it into Latin around 1552. The document is organised by ailment and features coloured drawings of the natural products, with labels of their Nahuatl names written in Spanish. Badiano was one of the students at the Colegio de Santa Cruz de Santa Cruz de Tlatelolco under the tutelage of Fray Bernardino de Sahagún. Students at the Colegio were selected from Nahua nobility and received a typical humanistic education: the trivium (grammar, logic and rhetoric) and the quadrivium (arithmetic, geometry, music and astronomy). In addition to becoming competent in Latin and Castilian, they also studied theology and religion. The Colegio was a short-lived experiment as increasingly over the colonial period a series of measures were put into place by Spanish authorities to limit Indigenous achievement in educational, religious and political arenas.

that today are fixtures of the colonial Latin American literary canon. But with Benavides, the author's interlocutors and companions are not primarily fellow explorers and soldiers, as with Cabeza de Vaca and his *Naufragios* [The Narrative of Cabeza de Vaca] (1542) or Bernal Díaz del Castillo's *Historia verdadera de la conquista de la Nueva España* (1551–84) [True history of the conquest of New Spain]. Rather, they are primarily men and women of varying ages and multiple backgrounds who are not as easily reduced to any one group. Benavides's difference in station, profession and situation compared to those of the authors whose testimonies have largely come to define what we think of as the European gaze in the case of encounter and early colonial literature leads him to notice other things and to privilege a different set of events, elements that may have been inconsequential in the context of a grand *historia* or a *relación*, allowing at times a more diverse set of period voices to come through.

The *Secretos* is the only book thought to have been written by Benavides. Very little is known about his biography, and most of what we do know about his life comes from the text itself, as no conclusive historical information has come to light about him.[21] He claimed to have been born in the Spanish city of Toro, in Zamora, perhaps around 1521. Despite being identified as 'doctor' on the title page and by the endorsing signatures, it is unlikely he had formal academic training, a conclusion supported by the need to acknowledge the presence of a supervising physician when performing certain medical procedures. His itinerary in the 1550s takes him first to the Canary Islands and, from there, to Santo Domingo, Honduras, Guatemala and finally to New Spain where he remained for eight years.[22] Although he mentions professional commitments sometimes required him to be absent from Mexico City, implying that his work involved a degree of mobility, it is likely he spent most of his time in the Mexican capital and may have worked at the Hospital de Amor de Dios given his expertise in the treatment of *bubas*, which that institution was known for. He alludes to other medical practitioners whose names appear in the historical record but his has not been found in any documents pertaining to the practice of medicine in the region.[23] The *Secretos* was written upon Benavides's return to Europe, where he obtained a licence for its publication in 1556, appearing in Valladolid a year later.

What kind of text is the *Secretos* and how are we to read it today? Already in his choice of title Benavides invited readers to place his work in the context of

21 See García Icazbalceta (1954, 231); Fresquet Febrer (1993, 17, 23–25); and Somolinos d'Ardois (1980a, 196–97).

22 Fresquet Febrer, following Somolinos d'Ardois, clarifies that the voyage must have taken place either in 1545 or in 1550, given that Benavides mentions being a travel companion of judge Zurita. If he departed from Spain with him, the voyage would date to 1545. If instead he joined him later, when he left New Granada for Santo Domingo, then the second date would stand (1993, 30).

23 Somolinos d'Ardois (1980, 196); Fresquet Febrer and López-Terrada (1999, 41).

'books of secrets', a corpus that by then enjoyed one of the longest traditions in Western popular literature, with the sixteenth century in particular being their heyday.[24] As William Eamon explains:

> The libri secretorum, or 'books of secrets,' were compilations of recipes, formulas, and 'experiments' of various kinds, including everything from medical prescriptions and technical formulas to magical procedures, cooking recipes, parlour tricks, and practical jokes. The one thing these assorted manuscripts had in common was the promise of providing access to the 'secrets of nature and art'. (1994, 16)

The *Secreta*, as they were known in Spain, arrived in Europe in the twelfth century, and quickly became one of the most widely circulated types of books of the Middle Ages. They trace their origins to the Hellenistic period and to the Roman encyclopaedic culture that strove to create ways of quickly accessing the fundaments of Aristotelian logic. Nonetheless, as Luis García Ballester points out, books of secrets 'required another type of knowledge different from Aristotle's; forms of knowledge that were not favoured by the establishment, which ended up preferring Aristotelian ideas' (2001, 63). Their true sources of information had more to do with the Hermetic tradition and with peripheral scientific literature and popular practices. Many such books purported to be direct testimonies of Aristotle without there being any truth to the claim when compared against the philosopher's known works.

As Elaine Leong and Alisha Rankin note, the notion of 'secret' in these texts can be understood as 'a set of procedures known only to a select group of initiated individuals—in other words, craft or trade secrets' which were 'more about technical know-how, or "how to" than hidden knowledge' (2011, 8). However, as Eamon clarifies, 'in the sixteenth century … the term was still densely packed with its ancient and medieval connotations' (1994, 5), giving Benavides's allusion to secrets at this point in time a wide semantic range. In the late fifteenth and early sixteenth centuries, the proliferation of books of secrets also led to their evolution. They began to concern themselves with new topics following the changing interests of European publics, turning to subjects like alchemy. The shift in focus is an important turn of events given that their fundamental premise had been to reveal 'new' information in the sense of re-establishing access to previously 'lost' information. Medieval *Secreta* had promised to reveal truths already discovered in Antiquity, but hidden or forgotten over time; to innovate had been, in fact, to restore. But the interest generated by greater accessibility to products arriving from the Far East, and then from the Americas, modified the conventions of the genre, which began to make way for themes outside the classical conceptual framework of the known world. While there would not be a body of 'New

24 For an overview of the rise in scholarship on books of secrets, see Leong and Rankin (2011, 1–20).

World *secreta*' as such, in addition to the *Secretos*, the term also made its way to one of New Spain's most important works on natural history published in 1591 by another physician, Juan de Cárdenas, the *Primera parte de los problemas y secretos marauillosos de las Indias* [First part of the problems and marvellous secrets of the Indies] to be examined over the course of the chapters that follow.

Like books of secrets, which not only discussed materials but emphasised methods and instructions, surgical manuals shared a similar interest in describing process. In the sixteenth century, surgeons were figures in between academic medical theory and daily practice. Although surgery was related to medicine, it was initially an extracurricular field of study that had developed largely on a separate plane. In Roman times, and later in the Middle Ages, good health was conceived in preventive terms, and medical knowledge focused predominantly on regimen as a means to regulate the interaction of the humours with other substances and with external conditions. Symptoms were the manifestation of the loss of that balance; if an illness arose, pharmaceutical as well as therapeutic treatments sought to restore the natural internal order that, once achieved, would result in the patient being healed or feeling well again. In contrast, surgery emerged as a last-resort treatment arising from the need to control haemorrhages in serious wounds or in cases of extreme or chronic pain. The kinds of surgical procedures that it was possible to perform with any expectation of success were restricted. Surgeons were careful not to attempt risky cures that would call into question their professional reputation or prolong the suffering of the patient. Vernacular medical treatises stressed the importance that the surgeon be capable of making this distinction, although it did not mean surgery was a rare or exceptional choice. The proliferation of surgical texts and the strong presence of surgeons in European societies suggest that, despite its limitations, as noted by Nancy Siraisi, 'the accomplishments of surgery satisfied prevailing social expectations' (1990, 158).

Surgery began to consolidate itself as a discipline during the eleventh century, thanks to the social and economic development of the period and to the discovery of Greek and Islamic materials that disseminated the ideas of figures like Celsus (second century AD) and Paul of Aegina (seventh century AD), the latter greatly influencing the work of Arab encyclopaedists such as Abū al-Qāsim Khalaf ibn 'Abbās al-Zahrāwī (Albucasis, tenth to eleventh centuries AD) and Ibn Sina (Avicenna, tenth to eleventh centuries AD), who played an important role in the development of medieval Spanish medicine. The twelfth- and thirteenth-century Latin translation of al-Zahrāwī's surgical treatises and of Ibn Sina's *Canon of Medicine* (1025) were read all over the continent; the *Canon* remained the most widely used text in Spanish universities until the Humanist reforms (Siraisi, 1990, 161). Often the dissemination of lengthy texts, full of specialised terminology, became fragmentary and inexact, prompting doctors and surgeons from the twelfth century on to assemble surgical compendia that facilitated access to information. Composed in vernacular languages or in Latin, their aim was to 'stimulate the reading of medical authorities and aid in learning medical concepts' (García Ballester, 2001, 347). These works, especially vernacular ones, sometimes took a life of their own outside strictly academic circles, and found their way to the hands of lesser medical practitioners alongside *florilegios* and recipe collections. Among the most widely read authors of this type of literature were Rogerius (twelfth century AD), Guglielmo da Saliceto (thirteenth century AD) and, in the fourteenth century, Guy de Chauliac, who would have a decisive impact on Spanish surgery, and on Benavides in particular. Chauliac's text was printed seven times in Spain before 1550, not including partial adaptations that also circulated as the *Flores de Guido* [Guido's flowers] (López Piñero, 1974, 59). The oral examination of Spanish surgeons would come to be based on the basic tenets of his work.

In his principal text, the *Inventarium sive Chirurgia Magna* (1363), Chauliac had offered a critical evaluation of the history of surgery, bemoaning the separation that he saw between the roles of the surgeon and the doctor. He defended the need to incorporate anatomical knowledge into surgical intervention, and complained that the precepts of Galenic and Hippocratic medicine were not taken into account in practice. Until Avicenna's time 'all were both physicians and surgeons', wrote Chauliac, but then 'surgery was separated [from medicine] and left in the hands of the mechanics' (1997, 298). The religious and political atmosphere in Spain exacerbated the separation between academic knowledge and medical circles that were excluded from the university. Important medical works had been written by *conversos* who faced a series of institutional obstacles to obtain formal titles.[25] Academic medicine towards the end of the fifteenth century and the beginning of the sixteenth century was preoccupied with regulating the labour of lesser medical practitioners, like surgeons, reflecting changing socio-religious attitudes. During the reign of the Catholic monarchs mechanisms of central supervision were established, such as the *Protomedicato*, which sought to define the roles of the various professions related to health. In the sixteenth century, surgery finally began to form part of institutional education in Spain, and the curricular reforms undertaken by Spanish universities led to the gradual inclusion of anatomy in their courses. Whereas 'only the University of Valencia [had] a permanent chair in anatomy' at the start of the century, as Bjørn Okholm Skaarup recalls in his in-depth study on anatomy in Spain during the early modern period, 'by the mid-1500s, similar permanent professorships had been established in Salamanca, Alcala de Henares, Coimbra and Barcelona' (2015, 30).[26]

25 García Ballester concluded that 'all the original medical production that we know of from Castile [in the fifteenth century] was written by doctors with university training, but not in the university' (2001, 316).

26 It should be noted that this trend did not continue into the seventeenth century. As Víctor Navarro observes, 'the overall decline of university education [in Spain] was

Perhaps the figure that best exemplifies the changing attitudes in European academic medicine which Benavides begins to articulate in the *Secretos* is Andreas Vesalius, who would become a physician at the Spanish court of Charles V and later of Philip II in the mid sixteenth century. Prior to this appointment, he had defended his lectureship in surgery and anatomy at the University of Padua before colleagues who questioned whether these fields were truly relevant to the study of medicine. In his landmark *De humani corporis fabrica libri septem* (1543), generally considered one of the most important medical texts ever printed and an immediate bestseller at the time of its publication, Vesalius had answered his critics in the following manner:

> When the whole practice of cutting was handed over to the barbers, not only did the physicians lose first-hand knowledge of the viscera, but also the whole art of dissecting fell forthwith into oblivion, simply because the physicians would not undertake to perform it, while they to whom the art of surgery was entrusted were too unlettered to understand the writings of the professors of anatomy. (1998, li)

Without making anatomical knowledge and dissection part of the education of doctors in a university context, dissections for Vesalius were a:

> detestable ritual whereby one group performs the actual dissection of a human body and another gives an account of the parts; the latter aloft on their chairs croak away with consummate arrogance like jackdaws about things they have never done themselves but which they commit to memory from the books of others or which they expound to us from written descriptions, and the former are so unskilled in languages that they cannot explain to the spectators what they have dissected but hack things up for display following the instructions of a physician who has never set his hand to the dissection of a body but has the cheek to play the sailor from a textbook. (1998, li)

Vesalius's use of navigation metaphors to characterise the task of the doctor who 'plays the sailor', is an example of how literature relating to anatomical dissection in the sixteenth century followed what Pedro Laín Entralgo calls the push for 'surgical invention as adventure ... comparing his activity with that of the navigators, conquistadors and great captains of the era'.[27] The inner body was seen as a new frontier, a *terra incognita*, and surgery as the

reflected in the fact that surgery, mathematics, and astronomy were among the seven chairs called "rare"—that is, uncommon, or exceptional—and often remained vacant' (2003, 321).

27 Laín Entralgo, cited in López Piñero (1998, 135). There are other examples of similar metaphoric language in early modern texts that sought to establish a positive association between the role of the medical practitioner and the figure of the Spanish explorer from earlier times. See Eamon's reading of the surgeon Giuseppe Zambeccari, who writes in the seventeenth century: 'I courageously embarked upon

liminal activity that allowed penetrating into the unknown. Benavides's case makes the image literal rather than metaphorical, fusing both roles, for here was a surgeon who wrote about his adventures as a medical professional and an overseas explorer.

While it could seem unusual for a medical work such as the *Secretos* to have a highly episodic character, its form finds precursors in the corpus of medieval surgical treatises that departed from other kinds of medical literature precisely on this point. According to Siraisi:

> One noteworthy feature of the surgeons' books is their willingness to tell stories about themselves, their patients, and their teachers, colleagues and pupils. Of course, the great bulk of surgical writing is not anecdotal; and anecdotes can also occasionally be found in other kinds of medical writing. Nonetheless, personal anecdote is markedly more prevalent in surgical than in other books. (1990, 170)

Benavides's text is divided into 79 chapters, a prologue, two endorsing signatures by doctors and surgeons Domingo de Cavala and Pedro de Torres, and a small list of errata that appears before the first chapter. Chapter 1, as well as chapters 24–45 are on *morbo gálico*, chapters 2–10 and 12–23 each centre on one medicinal ingredient, or 'simple' (mechoacan, guaiacum, maguey, guavas and others), chapter 11 is on the 'ailments of the Indies' but focuses primarily on a then deadly illness called the *chapetonada*, for it only afflicted 'chapetones' or Spaniards who had recently arrived in America and were derided with that moniker by locals, chapters 46–49 are on *mirrarchia*, chapter 50 is on fistulas of the penis, chapters 51–59 and 63–72 are on the treatment of wounds, chapters 60–62 are on eye problems, chapters 73–75 are on *lamparones*, chapters 76 and 77 discuss recommended compound medicines, chapter 78 is on how to treat injuries from a fall, and finally chapter 79 discusses how the text's findings have been vetted by 'learned men' [hombres doctos]. Despite the straightforward layout of the table of contents, the internal organisation of the material comes across as haphazard, relying on the author's own personal narrative and autobiography for a justification of the logic in the sequence of information shared.

Anecdotes and triumph over great challenges against the odds were a recurring theme in much of the exploration literature of the New World. Columbus, Cortés, Cabeza de Vaca and Díaz del Castillo all take the pen with aims very different from those of Benavides, yet they share in the elaboration of a self-referential and auto-historical discourse that brings events into focus from the point of view of personal experience, stressing the value of their own sacrifice in the defence of Spain's interests.[28] Benavides takes advantage of the shared sensibility between the medical treatise and early colonial

this [surgical procedure] exactly in the same way as the discoverers of the New World' (1994, 272).

28 See Merrim (1996, 58–100).

historiography, incorporating both. Without scenes of battle or capture, he will remind his readers of how he is one of just seven survivors of a transatlantic voyage that had seen 70 others perish (fols. 29v–30r), and how the knowledge accrued and shared in the book is not for his personal profit but for the greater glory of Spain, as adduced in the long title. As in medieval and renaissance surgical chronicles known to make use of the hagiographic model, Benavides—the surgeon—, appears at times as a figure under duress, whose ability and skill are being called into question by another character in the story. There is a curious transference of roles in surgical books, given that the surgeon was often risking life and limb, just not his own, with reputation rather than survival at stake. A surgeon's perseverance in the face of adversity—not challenges to chastity or faith but rather the dangers of incorrect treatments suggested by other characters (often female)—these were analogous to the martyr's temptations in the exempla. The final success of the surgeon's own proposed method elevated him as a chosen figure, marking the gulf between his insight and the ignorance of others, including less talented or less knowledgeable colleagues.

For example, one of the most detailed surgical cases narrated in the *Secretos* is that of a boy who had sustained a head injury that exposed the brain:

> Then kept in the heights of the church were some charged small culverins … A boy of thirteen arrived while one of the weapons was being fired. He turned his back and the muzzle recoiled backward, striking the boy in the head … I was called to treat the boy. I did so that day, finding he was unconscious. On the second day, they called another surgeon and a physician, and it was very bloody … the following day the bleeding relented, at which time I began to remove the pieces of bone. The next day, while removing more bone, out came a piece of wood, the size of half a fava bean, to which was attached a fragment of brain substance the size of half a chickpea, and let no one think this could have been sanies, for it was actual medullary substance.[29]

Although the reader fully expects that the outcome will be positive given the conventions of the surgical manual, the description of the incident nonetheless is spread over a chronological narrative structure that heightens a sense of suspense. The listing of choices made at every turn in the treatment are

29 'Tenían en lo alto de la iglesia unos versos cargados … y llegando un mozo de coro a pegar fuego a uno, volvió las espaldas y se abajó … y le alcanzó un pedazo de la cureña en la cabeza. Yo fui llamado para la cura, y le curé aquel día sin que él tuviese ningún sentido. A la segunda cura llamaron a otro cirujano y un médico, y había mucha sanguinolencia … Otro día siguiente nos dio lugar la sangre, empecé a sacar pedazos de huesos, y otro día sacando más huesos, salió tanto pedazo de bonete como grandeza de media haba, en el cual salió pegado tanta sustancia medular como medio garbanzo, y no piense nadie que esto fue sanies, sino que fue verdaderamente sustancia medular' (1567, fols. 121v–122r).

mixed with MacGuffin-esque details inconsequential to the cure, such as the exact manner of the weapon's discharge, or where ammunitions were kept. The narration also switches from the third person to the first person, drawing the focus away from the injured patient undergoing treatment to the author as the protagonist of the action. Precision comes by way of similes to familiar foodstuffs like chickpeas and fava beans, here related to size. And observations on the specific case in the passage are linked to larger statements about normative processes in the body and approaches to medical treatment:

> This being contrary to the Hippocratic aphorism, which states 'incisa vesica vel epate aud cor substantia cerebri penitus letale' [a wound exposing the bladder or the liver or the heart or brain is lethal], and the physician and the surgeon having seen the cerebral substance, they did not wish to continue with the cure, and since I was the first to arrive and the treatment was mine, I proceeded as best I could.[30]

The correct treatment is presented in opposition to an incorrect way of proceeding, which the reader is led to assume would have brought about the death of the patient. But the roles in this episode are not the same ones as one would expect in a surgical treatise. Benavides does not stand in opposition to an empiric or a meddling woman, who could be easily dismissed as ignorant, but against the figures of the doctor and the other surgeon, who function as intermediaries between the author and conventional Galenic medicine. The section underlines the contradiction between Benavides's leading role in administering emergency first-response care and the attention later received by the patient, even as it insists on the marginal place assigned to him when the other men arrive. In the context of the period, a mode of proceeding that contradicted the tenets of conventional humanistic medicine would not have been seen as innovative, but as ill-informed and risky, a public misstep into the intellectual terrain of the empirics that the doctor and other surgeon choose to avoid. 'Given the level of care available', remarks Fernando Chico, 'and the well-known poor outcomes for cases of severe head injuries, it would be the rare 16th century surgeon or physician who would even consider undertaking treatment in a clinical situation like [this] one' (2000, 218).[31] The rebellious challenge to hierarchical authority, familiar to readers

30 'Contra el aforismo de Hipócrates donde dice incisa vesica vel epate aud cor subtantia cerebri penitus letale y como el médico y el cirujano vieron la sustancia del cerebro no quisieron volver más a la cura. Y como yo había sido el primero, y la cura era mía, hube de ir prosiguiendo en ella, por el mejor estilo que yo pude' (1567, fols. 122r–122v).

31 Along with Fresquet Febrer's and Solomon's interventions already adduced, Chico's co-authored article is another recent scholarly output that has focused on Benavides and the *Secretos* specifically, but written from the disciplinary standpoint of present-day neurosurgery, and directed at medical professionals.

of the colonial Latin American canon, has more in common with gestures like Cabeza de Vaca's taking the reins at the failure in leadership of his superior Pánfilo de Narváez, or Cortés's rejection of Diego Velázquez's orders to halt the march towards Tenochtitlan compromising the momentum of the expedition, dressing the formula of the surgical treatise in the robes of New World accounts where an act of defiance is ultimately proven justified and recast as sanctioned, or even heroic.

The interweaving in the text of his lived experiences during the years spent away from Spain serve not only to structure the information that he gathers about diverse natural products, but also tell the tale of a developing subjectivity, at both personal and professional levels. Benavides offers himself as the only one for whom it was possible to act in such a manner and save the boy's life. His point of view, according to the *Secretos*, was unique, and, at least in this case, superior to that of those around him. On one hand, he had access to a record of experiences that fell outside the Galenic corpus. On the other, his readings allowed him to step in and out of that system. His eccentric position also afforded him a degree of protection, for in the event the patient did not survive, he could advance the position that death had come because of the type of injury sustained and the limitations of working in a colonial setting rather than as a result of his care. This was another advantage of including the Hippocratic aphorism, and of opting to leave it in Latin rather than translate it into Spanish, highlighting his level of linguistic competence and learned status even as he was performing the manual duties of a 'romance surgeon' or a barber.[32] Downplaying his treatment by characterising it as 'the best I was able to do', however, is countered by the length the narration devotes to the incident. The paradox deploys the rhetorical trope of *parvitas*, or false modesty, for in the pages that follow Benavides meticulously narrates the elements of the cure and the patient's prognosis. The first step had been to clean the wound, to then apply a mixture of emollients (mallow plant, egg whites and pink oil, among others) that disinfected as they anesthetised. Finally, he had covered the area with a cream made of beans to put pressure on the wound and help it heal. While he does not disclose it, the procedure and the ingredients he used reflect his readings and closely adhered to the techniques that had been advocated by both Chauliac and al-Zahrāwī in their texts, something that

32 The term 'cirujano romancista' was used to denote a medical practitioner whose training consisted primarily of an apprenticeship, and whose certification involved being examined by the Protomedicato in Castilian (a romance language) differentiating him from the 'cirujano latino' who could have some level of university education and who was examined in Latin. See Brouard Uriarte (1972, 239–53). The term is slippery, though, as sources most often use surgeon by itself, without making a clear distinction. Fresquet Febrer notices that there is no news of the aphorism quoted by Benavides in the known versions of works by Hippocrates, although he concedes it could be an unknown, lost version (1993, 155).

would have been apparent to any university-trained, physician-reader.[33] Yet despite the text-based origin of his method, the narration's emphasis at this juncture remains firmly on the author's own original observations and on his successful, self-guided decisions, opting to forego impressing the reader with intertextual references. Fresquet Febrer's analysis counts a total of 66 allusions to 24 medical sources (classical, medieval and of the period) in Benavides's book,[34] a very reduced number for a medical treatise, considering an author like Chauliac had included in his text over 3,500.[35] But in the *Secretos* what grants authority to a given remedy is not the allusion to a learned source but its habitual and effective use: 'I always cure with them' writes the Benavides of his medical techniques, 'and I proceed until the sore begins to form a scar.'[36] In the case of the youth's wound, Benavides's care proved remarkably effective: 'his name was Vergara', he boasts, 'and this was such a notorious event, that whoever you ask in Mexico about these affairs, will know it, and will tell you so'.[37]

Benavides's interest in highlighting the boy's story and the local fame it brought him was likely one of the ways in which he was trying to better position himself before the most influential of all sectors in Spanish society at the time upon his return to the continent: the monarchy. In 1562, then Crown prince don Carlos had suffered a fall resulting in a serious head wound. The accident had mobilised to his bedside all the major medical figures in Spain at the court of Philip II, including Vesalius, whose treatment advice would put him squarely at odds with the king's trusted medical entourage.[38] In the end, Vesalius's recommendations, which included invasive

33 According to Chico, Albucasis specified that if the cerebral membranes were visible 'it [was] convenient to separate the fragments and injured tissues ... first rasp the head wound to uncover the bone ... recover the wound with a pad soaked in wine and pink oil' (2000, 220). Chauliac for his part 'categorized head wounds into seven types and discussed the management of each in detail. ... He used egg albumin to stop bleeding and provide adequate hemostasis (always a difficult problem for surgeons to address), and this approach was also used by Dr. Arias' (Chico, 2000, 219).

34 The list includes 12 to Galen, 11 to Chauliac, nine to Giovanni da Vigo, four to Hippocrates, and three each by Avicenna and Ruiz Díaz de la Isla (Fresquet Febrer, 1993, 28).

35 According to Michael McVaugh in his edition of Chauliac, 'Guy's formation in the scholastic medical community is nowhere plainer than in the extraordinary frequency with which he makes use of citations and quotations from other authors to express his views. His sixteenth-century editors were so struck by this feature of the work that they listed his authorities and counted his references, enumerating 3.523 of them—and their count was in fact too low' (1997, xiii).

36 'yo curo siempre con ellas y procedo hasta que quiere cicatrizar la llaga' (1567, fol. 123r).

37 'El que yo curé se llamaba Vergara, esto fue cosa tan notoria, que a quien quiera de México que le pregunten estos casos, lo saben y lo dirán' (1567, fols. 124r–124v).

38 For an extended discussion on this event, see Skaarup (2015, 129–37).

measures and the handling of brain tissue, were not followed and don Carlos survived the ordeal by way of a less interventionist approach. The fact that the *Secretos* is dedicated to don Carlos is, therefore, doubly appropriate as an important figure whose case resembled Vergara's, and given the text's focus on the Americas in particular. During the reign of Charles V, several texts on the New World printed in Spain were either dedicated or addressed to then Crown Prince Philip II, who had been placed in charge of overseas affairs; there would have been a sense of continuity in repeating that gesture with the new Crown Prince, don Carlos. Surely Benavides hoped his work would resonate with the expected future monarch as well as with readers for whom accounts of dramatic head injuries would recall recent events. Unfortunately for him, it is unlikely that he received any benefit from his deference to don Carlos as the latter would die in 1568, shortly after the publication of the *Secretos*, under mysterious circumstances and in his father's disfavour. But while Benavides may have been unsuccessful in connecting with this particular reader, at least one of the surviving copies of the *Secretos* attests to its success with others.

Vernacular surgical books, not unlike conversion manuals, tended to be small in size, practical objects that served a referential function for private study but that could also be used in the field. As Michael Solomon observes, 'a medical treatise is a tool or instrument designed to assist the user, as would any quotidian object, such as a knife or sewing needle. Every instrument has the potential to suggest an idea (myth or fiction) of its implied function' (2010, 10). However, finding evidence that confirms the potential Solomon adduces tends to be a challenge for scholars, especially in the case of materials that are not amply cited by later sources, even if that absence does not preclude the possibility that a given text enjoyed wide use. 'The copies of Renaissance texts that have survived', explains William H. Sherman, 'represent only a fraction of those that were produced; and the more heavily a book was used, the more vulnerable it was to decay' (2008, 5). The problem is sometimes further confounded by nineteenth-century binding practices, which would trim imprints, destroying information like firebrands or marginalia, and could go as far as bleaching printed materials to rid them of 'scribbling'. In this context, Benavides's case provides an extraordinary window into a relationship that is usually extremely difficult to recuperate in the early modern archive.

Placed next to period anatomical sources like Vesalius's *Fabrica* or Juan Valverde de Amusco's *Historia de la composición del cuerpo humano* [Anatomy of the human body] (1556), the *Secretos*'s medical illustrations may seem crude or unimpressive. And yet they perform a task that eludes the images in these works by closing the gap between the metaphorical potentiality of a medical book that becomes a tool in an embodied experience. There are three illustrations in the *Secretos*, one of a surgical incision, one for use in an invasive, non-surgical procedure and one of a medical instrument. The illustration in folio 92r (see figure 1.2) relates to the treatment of *bubas* and

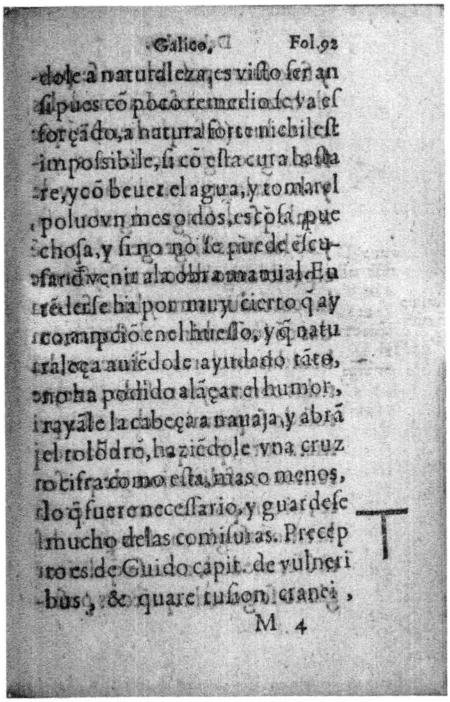

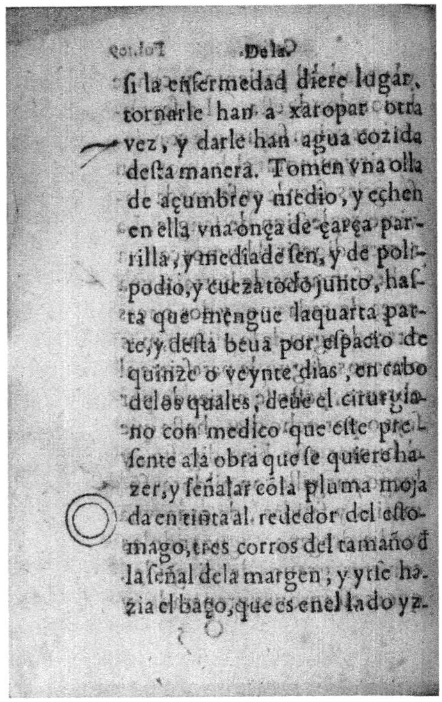

Figures 1.2a and 1.2b. True-to-life-sized images of surgical incisions in folio 92r and of a cutaneous mark in folio 109v of the *Secretos*. The image in the shape of a capital T is for cranial bloodletting in the treatment of *bubas* (left), and the circular pattern is for a gastrointestinal invasive treatment, to be drawn seven times on the patient's torso at the height of the stomach, towards the spleen (right). Courtesy of the US National Library of Medicine.

accompanies a passage instructing the reader to 'shave [the patient's] scalp with a razor, and open the tumour with a cross or sign like this one, more or less, adapting it to what is necessary'.[39] The image in folio 109v was for use in the treatment of *mirrarchia*: 'With a physician present to perform this task', directs Benavides, 'the surgeon should draw with a plume dipped in ink three circles around the patient's stomach the size indicated on the margin, toward the spleen, which is on the left side, under the ribs.'[40] The instructions continue by asking the surgeon to draw four more circles.

39 'ráyenle la cabeza a navaja, y ábranle el golondro, haciéndose una cruz o cifra como ésta, más o menos, lo que fuere necesario' (1567, fol. 92r).

40 'debe el cirujano con médico que esté presente a la obra que se quiere hacer, y señalar con la pluma mojada en tinta alrededor del estómago, tres corros del tamaño de la señal del margen, e irse hacia el bazo, que es en el lado izquierdo, debajo de las costillas' (1567, fols. 109v–110r).

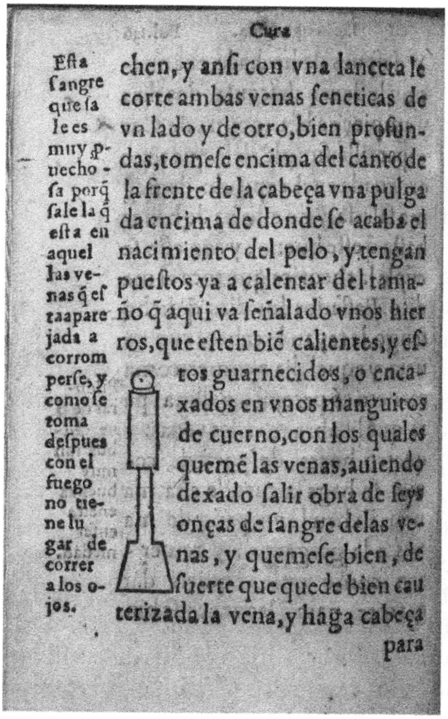

Cura

Eſta ſangre que ſale es muy provechoſa porq ſale la q eſta en aquel las venas q eſtaaparejada a corromperſe, y como ſe toma deſpues con el fuego no tiene lugar de correr a los ojos.

chen, y anſi con vna lanceta le corte ambas venas ſeneticas de vn lado y de otro, bien profundas, tomeſe encima del canto de la frente de la cabeça vna pulgada encima de donde ſe acaba el nacimiento del pelo, y tengan pueſtos ya a calentar del tamaño q aqui va ſeñalado vnos hierros, que eſten bie calientes, y eſtos guarnecidos, o encaxados en vnos manguitos de cuerno, con los quales queme las venas, auiendo dexado ſalir obra de ſeys onças de ſangre delas venas, y quemeſe bien, de ſuerte que quede bien cauterizada la vena, y haga cabeça para

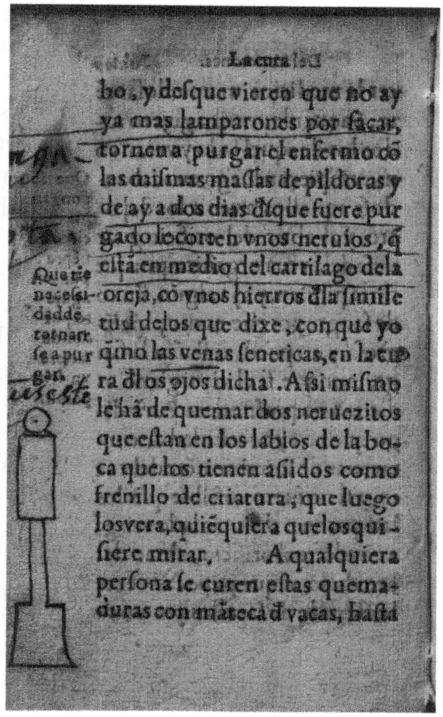

La cura

Que tiene neceſsidad de tornarſe a purgar.

bo, y deſque vieren que no ay ya mas lamparones por ſacar, tornen a purgar el enfermo cō las miſmas maſſas de pildoras y de ay a dos dias dſque fuere purgado le corten vnos neruios, q eſtā en medio del cartilago dela oreja, cō vnos hierros dla ſimilitud delos que dixe, con que yo q̄mo las venas ſeneticas, en la cura dlos ojos dicha. Aſsi miſmo le hā de quemar dos neruezitos que eſtan en los labios de la boca que los tienen aſidos como frenillo de criatura, que luego los vera, quiē quiſiera que los quiſiere mirar. A qualquiera perſona ſe curen eſtas quemaduras con māteca d vacas, haſta

Figures 1.3a and 1.3b. Folio 136v of the *Secretos* with Benavides's design for an instrument intended to cauterise blood vessels in the eye (left), and folio 159v of the British Library's copy of the book, showing where a reader has hand drawn the image from the earlier folio next to a different passage that again mentioned the device (right). Image of fol. 136v courtesy of the US National Library of Medicine. Image of fol. 159v used by permission of the British Library, digitised by Google, Digital Store 1607/102.

White-hot cauterising tools 'should be then placed on the marks previously made on the gut, and with those tools there is no need to cut'.[41] Benavides's explanation that they are not only accurate in shape, but true to life in size, turns the page into an object designed to be used physically on the surface of the body, overtaking Solomon's metaphorical divide. A similar process occurs with the third image found in folio 136v, this time, of an instrument designed to be used in the treatment of *optalmia*, a chronic illness that caused tumours in the eyes (see figure 1.3a). To eliminate them, Benavides used a hot iron with which he burned and cauterised the veins

41 'asienten [los hierros] sobre las señales que están hechas en la barriga, y con aquellos hierros no hay necesidad de penetrar' (1567, fol. 110r).

that furnish blood to the diseased structure, leading them to wither and fall off. Images of medical tools appeared in a number of anatomical sources of the period, including Vesalius's *Fabrica* which featured a woodcut devoted specifically to his collection of dissection tools, displayed strewn on top of a table with indexical labels identifying each one. However, despite the *Fabrica's* attention to detail, the image in the *Secretos* is arguably more precise in that it conveys an exact shape and size template to the reader in a way that Vesalius does not.

Print illustrations in medical books tend to remain but invitations into our reconstruction of plausible processes. Without additional information, it is difficult to determine if surgical and anatomical illustrations informed actual practice in addition to serving a referential function. Two copies of the *Secretos* are housed at Spain's National Library and show minor signs of use (some underlining and manicules).[42] The copy at the National Library of France has underlining and summarises some sections in the margins, like the one on *morbo gálico*. The copy at the National Library of Medicine (US), while amply annotated with crosses, does not bring us closer to answering the question of whether (or how) readers used these materials. But the copy at the British Library (UK), while unable to confirm that Benavides's design crossed over from a representation of an object into a physical one built to his specifications, does confront us with evidence of a reader who created his or her own visual object modelled after the print image. In a later section of the text concerning abscesses resulting from *scrofula*, Benavides's prose alludes to the tool shown in the earlier chapter on *optalmia*, explaining it could also be used to sever nerves in the outer ear, to which a reader of this particular copy responded by drawing in the same image as marginalia. So exact is the manner of the sketch compared to the original illustration that it almost fails to register as a manuscript annotation, opening a space that chronicles not only the author's experience, but the reader's as well (see figure 1.3b).

Indeed, narrating experience at times seems to become the more important consideration for Benavides. The section on avocados, for example, begins by touting these fruits as being 'very medicinal', and particularly good for the elderly since they are soft on toothless gums and are also a favourite choice due to their due to their taste. Benavides is emphatic on this point stating that the elderly 'go crazy for it' [mueren por ella] (1567, fol. 49r). But the passage soon veers into a consideration of those 'who affirm it is very powerful, and very useful to human generation'.[43] While at first it seems the author will let the oblique mention of the avocados' aphrodisiac properties suffice, going on to a meticulous description of ways to prepare them for consumption, the narration is drawn back to information of dubious surgical relevance:

42 One of the BNE's copies is incomplete, missing the last two chapters. For more on manicules and marginalia in early modern texts see Sherman, 2008, 34.

43 'dicen y afirman ser muy potencial, y muy provechosa, a la generación humana' (1567, fols. 49r–49v).

> They have a saying in those parts, 'avocados, father', and the reason for it is there was once a man who was very poorly, and [speaking to a priest who] enquired about the reason for his illness, and whether it had been caused by excesses with a woman, he responded that yes, [he had been with her] a great deal many times in a short period, and querying him once again to ask if he had done anything to bring about the sex act, he replied that he had eaten many avocados, and to all those who asked him, in his very weakened state, he would answer: 'avocados, father', and thus the saying arose.[44]

Although the saying does not survive in present-day Spanish usage, it does appear in sources other than Benavides's text, captured also in Gonzalo Correas's *Vocabulario de refranes y frases proverbiales* [Vocabulary of sayings and proverbial phrases], a project compiled in Spain around 1627.[45] By that point in time, and now in a European rather than New World context, the story had acquired additional resonances that poked fun at Church officials and that reconfigured the race and the gender of the 'weak man', substituting him for a lust-driven and shrewd *mulata* woman instead.[46]

Avocados are mentioned by many early New World chroniclers, including Pedro Cieza de León, Fernández de Oviedo, Alonso de Molina, and Martín Fernández de Enciso, who was especially taken with them and whose *Suma de geographia* [Collection on geography] published in Seville in 1519 was possibly the first European source to introduce them to overseas readers.[47] Called 'perales' because of their resemblance to pears by some sources

44 'tienen por refrán aguacates padre, y fue por esta razón que un hombre estaba muy malo, y preguntándole la causa de su enfermedad, y si había procedido de tener exceso con alguna mujer, repondió que sí, gran cantidad de veces en poco tiempo, y repreguntándole si había hecho alguna cosa para el coito repondió que había comido muchos aguacates, y a cuantos le preguntaban respondía, con la gran flaqueza que tenía, aguacates padre y a esta causa quedó el refrán dicho' (fols. 50r–50v).

45 Correas's text did not appear in print at the time, but it did circulate throughout the seventeenth and eighteenth centuries, used to supplement other projects. It would be printed eventually in its entirety by the Real Academia in 1906.

46 The version in the *Vocabulario* reads: 'Avocados, Father. They are fruits from the Indies, conducive to lust, as are here pine nuts, or snails, or Spanish fly. As she was confessing her sins, a *mulata* woman made it a point to mention having eaten avocados for a certain occasion, and during her account, and at its end, the confessor asked many times what fruit it was she had eaten so he could better remember it; and she would respond: "Avocados, father", so much so that she began to wonder why [the priest] was so keen to know, and whether he did not have other motives for his interrogation' (Correas, 2000, 49). Martha Lilia Tenorio also notices this passage in Correa and analyses it in the context of colonial poetic language; see Tenorio (2010, 347–402).

47 Although Fernández de Enciso does not give them a name, his description is especially emphatic on their quality: 'what they have inside is like butter and is of marvellous flavor and leaves a taste so good and soft that it is a marvellous thing'

early on, as well as 'paltas' from the Quechua term 'paltay' in regions further south, Benavides uses 'aguacates', a term derived from the Nahuatl's 'ahuacatl' which also meant testicles and, according to some scholars, was already considered an aphrodisiac in Nahua medicine before the arrival of Europeans.[48] However, the reasons for including avocados in the context of the textual economy of the *Secretos* are unclear for, unlike other New World herbs and plants that had begun to make their way to overseas botanical gardens, there is little evidence of attempts to grow these fruits in Europe until much later in the eighteenth century. If efforts had been made to introduce them by fellow returning travellers, they certainly had not been successful enough by the time of the text's publication to make avocados part of a reliable pharmaceutical supply.[49] Why does a presumably pragmatic surgical treatise then devote such attention to an American medicinal product that health practitioners in Valladolid would likely never have at their disposal? Instead of shying away from content that remained outside the scope of his European readers' reach, the *Secretos* often moves in the opposite direction, embracing its literary function and taking pleasure in narrating experiences chronicling life overseas in colonial communities. These digressions tend to be successfully incorporated into observations of scientific value, but they are made subordinate to narrative aims in ways that highlight a sense of continuity with writing about the New World at the time.

One such case is the section on *tunas*, alluding to an unspecified variety of prickly pear. The mention of *tunas* became a staple anecdote and running joke in early Spanish exploration texts and colonial-era literature, even though the fruit itself remained elusive in Europe. Variations of the same vignette told with different degrees of humour are found in sources as wide ranging as the texts penned by Fernández de Oviedo, Francisco López de Gómara, Francisco Cervantes de Salazar, and even Inca Garcilaso de la Vega in the first decade of the seventeenth century. Benavides's own version reads as follows:

> Many tricks have been played with the *tunas* on the newly arrived doctors in the following manner. Someone decides to eat many of these fruits, and then urinates in a receptacle, and takes the urine to him [the doctor], which is the colour of fresh blood, and the doctor orders many cooling remedies, and some phlebotomies, and the one who has the urine, or him to whom it belongs, says very discretely: let us leave this matter for today

['lo que tienen de dentro es como manteca y es de maravilloso sabor y deja el gusto tan bueno y tan blando que es cosa maravillosa'] (1519, fol. 66v).

48 Gómez de Silva explains that 'ahuacacuahuitl' translated as 'the testicles tree, given that it was used as an aphrodisiac' (2004, 6).

49 The earliest news of avocados being grown successfully locally date to the late eighteenth century, mentioned in the context of the Botanical Garden of Orotava in Tenerife, an institution in the Canary Islands which had been founded in 1791 with the purpose of acclimating overseas natural products to Europe. See Hernández González and Prieto Pérez (2007, 221).

> and tomorrow, for I am very much an enemy of medicines, and if things get worse, I shall send for you, sir. And the following day the doctor comes calling, and he tells him: sir, without doing anything whatsoever the illness has gone away. And the doctor is left fearful and terrified. These and other such tricks are played on the new doctors that arrive in the Indies. And the *indianos vaquianos*[50] (which means the older settlers) have as a rule not to call for any doctor until they have known him for two years, because they want these newly arrived doctors [coming from Spain], who are mostly young men, to first gather experience of things relating to medicine on others and not on them.[51]

While in other versions of this story the newcomer is tricked into consuming one of the fruits himself without knowing its effects so that others can laugh at his distress upon thinking he is passing blood instead of urine, in Benavides's text the horror comes not at the thought of the subject's fears of his own impending death from haemorrhage, but as a result of Eurocentric certainties being turned upside down in the New World. Benavides makes the medical case into a larger reflection on epistemology and the value of being sensitive to an American geographic setting as well as issues pertaining to experience and age. The single anecdote becomes a lead-in to remarks about the general mores of the settlers who resist being treated as if they were 'conejillos de Indias' [Guinea pigs] to use the phrase *avant la lettre*.[52] They care little about the doctors' qualifications or prior

50 According to María Elvira Sagarzazu, following Corominas, 'baquiano' came from the Arabic *baquîya*, meaning 'the rest, or what remains', and notes it was used by several colonial era sources including Fernández de Oviedo, Acosta and Inca Garcilaso (113).

51 'Con las tunas coloradas han hecho muchas burlas a médicos nuevos recién idos allá de esta manera. Come uno muchas de aquellas tunas, y orina en un orinal, y llévale la orina, y es como sangre viva, y el médico manda hacer muchos remedios refrigerativos, y algunas flebotomías, y el que tiene la orina, o cuya es, dice muy disimuladamente, dejémoslo por hoy y mañana, que soy muy enemigo de medicinas, y si fuere la cosa adelante yo llamaré a vuestra merced, y otro día adelante viénele el médico a visitar, y dice, señor sin hacerle nada se me ha quitado, y el médico está atemorizado y espantado. Estas, y otras burlas semejantes hacen a los médicos nuevos, que van a las Indias, y los indianos vaquianos en la tierra (que quiere decir viejos) en las Indias, tienen por estilo de no se curar con médico ninguno, hasta que haya pasado dos años por ellos, que quieren primero que estos tales médicos recién idos, que por la mayor parte son mozos hagan experiencia de las cosas tocantes a las medicinas en otros, y no en ellos' (1567, fols. 45r–46r).

52 The phrase 'Guinea pigs' or 'conejillos de Indias' (literally 'rabbits from the Indies' in Spanish) would not be used with the meaning it has today until the nineteenth century, even though the animals were used in medical experiments at least as far back as the eighteenth century. They were imported into Europe already in the sixteenth century subsequently becoming popular as pets. It is evocative that the expression used to convey the sense of an available and disposable (animal) body to

studies, which are not brought up, and more about a proven record of successful professional performance that they could observe first-hand. The newly arrived doctors are young still; it is but a laugh and they are given the chance to redeem themselves. Tellingly, it is a process that also hints at the need to become a part of the local community by spending two years becoming acquainted with their potential patients; a timed process of social and cultural acclimation.

The section acquires a wider resonance in the *Secretos* as Benavides provides a counterbalance in another episode on a newly arrived physician who, unlike the other group of inexperienced doctors, does enjoy a more privileged position within the medical establishment. He is judged more harshly:

> A very famous doctor, who went [there from Spain], fell ill with this illness of dysentery, and he was so arrogant and pleased with his own ability that even before arriving in Mexico while still in Our Lady of Guadalupe, which is one league away from Mexico City, he began to threaten doctors and surgeons … When he arrived in the Indies, he ate many bad local fruits, and fell ill with choleric dysentery, and trusting his own ability as I have said, although some local doctors[53] advised him of what he should do, and certified to him the customary progression of that illness in that land, he responded: 'Be gone your lordships with God', accusing them of wanting to kill him. And he prepared a bath, with cold water up to his stomach, and being so frail he died in it, and was left full of [his] medicines and remedies, because he did not wish to employ the ones that were used in the land.[54]

be used for research retains an association with European colonial settings (Africa and America) in both languages. For a more detailed account of Europe's interest in guinea pigs and scientific endeavours, see Endersby (2007, 212–19).

53 Benavides uses the phrase 'médicos de la tierra', which suggests that they are not only local doctors but specifically physicians of Indigenous descent rather than settled Europeans. The phrase 'gente con mezcla de la tierra' appears in at least one other period text from New Spain with the sense given to the word *mestizo* in colonial documents (see chapter 2).

54 'Un médico muy famoso, que fue de España, le dio esta enfermedad de cámaras, y él iba tan soberbio, y satisfecho de su habilidad, que antes que llegase a México empezó [a] amenazar a médicos y a cirujanos, estando en Nuestra Señora de Guadalupe, que es [a] una legua de México … Como abordó a las Indias, él comió muchas frutas malas de la tierra, y diéronle unas cámaras coléricas, y él fiándose en su habilidad (como dicho tengo aunque hubo algunos médicos de la tierra que le aconsejaron lo que debía hacer [y] le certificaron los sucesos de aquella enfermedad en aquella tierra, y él les respondía, váyanse vuestras mercedes con Dios, que si le querían matar, y así se metió en una tina de agua fría hasta el estómago, y como estaba tan descuidado salió de allí muerto, y quedó lleno de medicinas y remedios de ellas, porque no quiso hacer ninguna de las que se usaban en la tierra' (1567, fols. 52v–53v).

It is the arrogance and lack of foresight on the part of the European physician rather than his inexperience as a practitioner or the nature of the illness that causes his downfall. After all, Benavides had once also been a newcomer to the New World in his own right, and he too had suffered the so-called 'chapetonada' when he first arrived in Mexico, landing him at death's door.[55] But he had overcome this disadvantage both scientifically and socially—the running theme linking his professional and personal life in the *Secretos* when read as Benavides's memoir. He firmly establishes a rhetorical distance between his own open-minded attitude and that of a different kind of newly arrived European physician. In the case of the 'very famous' (albeit unnamed) doctor, Benavides does not recognise himself in his fellow countryman; he appropriates his colleague's voice in the first person for an instant ('váyanse vuestras mercedes con Dios') only to highlight his lack of self-control and ridicule him to cruelly comic effect. In the guise of a cautionary tale, the literary characterisation of the doctor becomes a fable caricature of those who fail to acknowledge the value of local resources, both medicinal (the remedies) and human (the advice of the local doctors).

The *Secretos* opens a discursive space for what Foucault terms a new 'enunciative modality'[56] that shares in the strategies of colonial-era *criollo* discourse, but it does so before this platform has been fully articulated as such, and importantly, without making it contingent upon birthplace. On the whole, Benavides does not seem invested in clarifying whether the people portrayed in the text as local are European or American-born, nor is there an explicit exclusion either of people of Indigenous descent from a common vantage point setting them apart from others who are shown as outsiders. Case in point, was Vergara a first generation *criollo* (as Spaniards born in America would come to be known)? Or given his last name, was he a Guipuzcoa native, from the continent but brought to the New World as a child? Could he have been a *mestizo*? Was he one of the many Indigenous youth living in Mexico City who had been baptised with a Christian name? The *Secretos* does not say; what matters in the text is that he was well known in New Spain, and that it had been Benavides's medical skill that had saved his life. Physical presence rather than point of origin, accumulated professional experience that was receptive toward innovation, appreciation of one's surroundings and successful integration within one's community are all presented as pathways to social belonging. The treatment of the figure of

55 The 'mal de cámaras' was a common gastrointestinal ailment that afflicted many Europeans that traveled to the New World, mentioned in numerous medical texts. According to the *Tesoro* (1611), the origin of the term comes from its association with the domestic space, 'being a thing that one does hiding and separately, it was called *cámara* [chambers], as the place one purges the abdomen is called *privada* [private] and *letrina* [from the Latin *lavatrina*, or washbasin], being done privately and hiding' (Covarrubias, 1998, 275).

56 See Foucault, 2002, 124.

the stubborn physician anticipates controversies that come to a head during the colonial period between *criollos* and *peninsulares* (Spaniards born in the continent) but it does not map onto it exactly. We find the seeds of what Jorge Cañizares-Esguerra in an eighteenth-century context has called 'patriotic epistemology', an intellectual stance that stressed 'the limited ability of outsiders to ever comprehend the history of America and its peoples', and that also made frequent use of humour and mockery (2001, 8).[57] But at this earlier juncture, in the mid sixteenth century, the criteria by which that line is drawn allowed for what may seem to us now a paradoxical position: European-born authors claiming insider status while reserving the right to adjudicate outsider status to others at their discretion. To put it another way, the 'Spaniards of the Indies', as Juan de Cárdenas would call them in his own writing, even as they begin to express a sense of allegiance to a new geographic space, had not yet realised they would not be allowed to be simply Spaniards, fully partaking of that identity label regardless of whether they lived in Spain or elsewhere. The difference between Europeans born abroad and those born in Europe was still a matter of circumstance rather than substance (as will be discussed in chapter 2). Someone like Benavides could find himself at home in the multi-ethnic but to him still familiarly European community of New Spain in the mid sixteenth century, and felt entitled to single out those whose attitudes precluded their inclusion within it.

As with several cornerstone texts in the colonial Latin American literary canon, the experiences narrated in the *Secretos* are mediated by time, written after the fact and, in Benavides's case, also by place. His use of 'here' and 'there' place him squarely in Europe from a geographical standpoint: 'there' will always mean 'in the Indies'. Likewise, in keeping with the discursive position usually adopted by the authorial voice in period medical texts, Benavides uses the first person singular (that is, 'I' rather than 'we') to mark his own discursive platform, referring to other figures in the third person (he, she, they), irrespective of whether they shared his gender or ethnicity. And yet, the physical displacement his journey entailed, and the network of relationships built over the years with social and physical surroundings, arguably recalibrated his critical vantage point to a set of coordinates different from those of the book's immediate audience. He may have been a Spanish author, living back in Spain, writing a book for fellow Spaniards, but what he created instead with the *Secretos* was in many ways an American text, one that turned Valladolid into a satellite site of early colonial enunciation.

57 According to Cañizares-Esguerra: 'In the discourse of patriotic epistemology, the foreign observer appeared as nemesis of learned clerical witness. Foreign travelers were portrayed as helpless victims of Amerindian cunning, who in any case paid only short visits to the lands they studied and were therefore unable to discover much about them. … Travelers were at the mercy of communities that gulled foreigners and laughed at their expense' (2001, 208). On this point, see also Goodman, 2009, 24–29.

Over the next decades, intellectuals in Mexico and Peru would unwittingly echo Benavides, especially in his critique of Seville's monopoly on information about the New World, and in challenging the peripheral role they were increasingly assigned in a transatlantic framework of scientific knowledge production, targeting some of the same figures, like Monardes, whose voice continued to overshadow theirs.[58] For its part, after its only known edition, the *Secretos* would slip into obscurity, another minor surgical text awash in the vast corpus of scientific and medical literature of Europe as it inched closer to the so-called Scientific Revolution. One copy of the book is listed in the 1573 inventory of the Marquis de Astorga's library,[59] but no other details about its fate with European readers have come to light thus far. However, in a promissory note dated 21 July 1576 from a certain Pablo García, a resident of Mexico City, to Alonso Losa, a local bookseller at the viceregal capital who traded in imports, we find an order request for the purchase of 'two Secretos de Cirugia [valued each at] one peso – two pesos total'.[60] Benavides most likely never returned to New Spain or to the Americas, but at least we know his book made it home.

58 As Daniela Bleichmar observes, Monardes was 'practically the only European source of information on New World *materia medica*' and 'for fifty years after the *Historia medicinal* appeared ... the major European authority on the uses of New World products to treat a wide range of medical conditions' (2005, 85–87).

59 See Cátedra (2002, 206).

60 See Leonard (1992, 205, 341).

CHAPTER 2

Irreconcilable differences?

Anatomy, physiology and the New World body

Information about American medicinal products as well as illness began flowing into Europe, dispersed in a variety of sources, almost immediately following Columbus's first voyages to the Caribbean.[1] Although not usually the main focal point in the early accounts of explorers, soldiers or religious men, there would be a rising interest in the topic of medicine as the century wore on, both in European and Mexican sources. In the case of print outputs, these varied considerably in scope and form, from personal travel narratives not unlike those of conquistador figures, to surgical manuals that mentioned Indigenous remedies, to formally structured volumes on *materia medica* and natural history. Especially in the case of materials written by authors with a humanist background and who had the chance to travel outside Europe, some not only attempted to reconcile long-standing Greco-Roman ideas about health, such as humoral theory, with new scientific knowledge, but they also devoted a significant portion of their texts to narrative prose, recounting personal experiences that mixed scientific appraisals with biography and social commentary, highlighting for readers the novelty of their situation as observers living and working in a non-Western setting.[2]

1 A helpful resource to trace the circulation of news about American natural products is the co-authored *Medicinas, drogas y alimentos vegetales del Nuevo Mundo* (1992), in which the authors in which the authors collate the passages that first mentioned them in European sources. While some of Noble David Cook's claims in his 1993 article on the spread of pathogens from Europe to the New World need to be updated in light of more recent findings in medical anthropology and epidemiology, his analysis remains a key source to understand the factors at play in the transmission of diseases from Europe to America between 1492 and 1518. For a discussion on Columbus's shifting views about the Caribbean as a healthy environment in his first voyage to a place harmful to Europeans' health, see Pérez Marín (2011).

2 Although the present study focuses on naturalists and medical writers associated with New Spain, Garcia da Orta's *Coloquios dos simples e drogas he cousas mediçinais da India*, published in Goa in 1563, and Cristóbal Acosta's *Tractado Delas Drogas, y medicinas de las Indias Orientales*, published in Burgos in 1578 (and largely based on Orta's work) exhibited similar tendencies, venturing beyond medical issues into

As seen in the previous chapter with the figure of Benavides, the physical displacement that turned an otherwise sedentary figure like the European medical practitioner into an errant observer of foreign lands could result in the writing of texts that did not quite fit the mould. A surgical treatise stretched its limits to make way for extended asides on the vicissitudes of travel, or a chapter purporting to focus on a straightforward discussion of a chronic ailment veered off topic into humorous anecdotes that only tangentially related to the medical issue at hand. An experience abroad had the potential to change the contents and structure of a medical text in this way, and it also had the power to open an analytical space for comparative assessments where Iberian understandings on matters like ethnic difference could be relativised and realigned to more immediate concerns being felt in colonial arenas. During the second half of the sixteenth century, anatomy and physiology would both seek to outline the contours of a normative body. But whereas in anatomy the push would be to minimise variation by proposing a template largely—albeit not completely—informed by successive confirmation, physiology would advance the idea of different bodies whose characteristics and capacities relied on their environments and their place within a given *nación*. The latter approach conflated emerging notions of ethnic background and racial identity with language that in later periods would be associated with taxonomical categories and biological determinism.

In Andalusia during the last quarter of the sixteenth century, Navarrese physician and author Juan Huarte de San Juan in his *Examen de ingenios para las ciencias* [The examination of men's wits] (1575), a bestseller that became a landmark source on natural philosophy and science of the early modern era, began to discuss human variation in a predominately Ibero-centric way. Huarte volunteered an appraisal of the bodies and minds of different European groups compared with one another, and in relation to populations in Africa, Asia and the Middle East, all this, as in Monardes's case, from information gleaned without venturing outside Spain.[3] His book associated the distinguishing characteristics of various groups with a number of positive value judgments, but the *Examen* was not a celebration of difference. It was a treatise that organised aptitudes qualitatively and yet hierarchically, with

descriptions of life in new colonial settings. Ines G. Županov observes that period audiences also remarked on this trend as not conforming to expectations, noting that one of the endorsing signatures in the *Coloquios* asked readers to excuse Orta for 'sometimes mov[ing] away from medicinal topics and relat[ing] some things of this country which are worth knowing' (Liçenciado Dimas Bosquet, cited in Županov, 2010, 45). Županov notes, however, that as in the case of Benavides, '[w]herever Orta's ethnographical digression takes us, we return in the end to the body' (2010, 45).

3 The *Examen* would be translated into English, Italian, Dutch, French and German, and was read by figures ranging from Francis Bacon, Inca Garcilaso de la Vega, Francisco de Quevedo and Lope de Vega all the way to Immanuel Kant, Arthur Schopenhauer and Fredrich Nietzsche in later periods.

membership in some groups being more desirable than others, reifying period attitudes toward race and class.

Huarte drew lines in the sand between *naciones* in a manner that increasingly brings us closer to modern racial labels, feeding what has proven to be a remarkably resilient model on the limits of normative Iberianness, one that obscured the Peninsula's own ethnically diverse past, and that all but negated the likely reality of centuries of miscegenation, unevenly distributed across that geographic territory depending on the socio-historical specificity of a given city or region. As Peter Wade's work on the links between modern genomics and notions of race clarifies, 'in the pursuit and maintenance of hierarches of value and power, relative purities are carved out of the sea of mixtures, by dint of selective genealogical tracings of particular connections, the enforcement of categorical distinctions, and exclusive practices', adding that 'what is seen as pure for some purposes can be understood as mixed for others; behind every purity, a mixture can be revealed with sufficient digging' (2017, 4).[4] Refashioning humoral theory through the lens of physical appearance and geographic origin, in the *Examen* Huarte had argued that different *naciones* of men possessed different intrinsic qualities that in turn explained disparities in aptitudes and intelligence levels:

> And experience it self-evidently shows this, how different are the Greeks from the Scythians, and the French from the Spanish, and the Indians from the Germans, and those from Ethiopia from the English. And this may be seen not only in regions that are far from one another, but if we consider the provinces around all of Spain we can distribute virtues and vices, … let us consider the wit and the mores of Catalans, Valencians,

4 For an extended discussion on how modern genomic science portrays contextual ideas on race informed by colonial terminology see Wade, 2017. Scholarship analysing current methods used by for-profit companies making scientific claims on racial categories for commercial ends remains a necessary but largely outstanding endeavour. Research on what companies like Ancestry.com term 'consumer genetics' has begun to look at problems with relying on statistically dominant DNA profiles of living, present-day subjects in a given region to make claims about ancestral origin and national belonging, particularly in diverse early modern settings with several groups of long-standing ethnic minorities (see, for example, the description of the Illumina OmniExpress platform for genotyping in 'Ancestry DNA Ethnicity Estimate White Paper' as well as Ancestry's 'Iberian Identity' page). Likewise, new interdisciplinary research has begun to challenge the scientific basis on which markers and loci are selected when estimating genetic clustering (see Blell and Hunter, 2019). Further studies could investigate more fully the implications of the marketisation of genealogy in the context of corporate models where scholarly expertise on cultural studies, migration studies, medieval and early modern history and area studies is not usually represented at a high level in a company's workforce, or at one that matches the investment in 'scientists with backgrounds in population genetics, statistics, machine learning, and computational biology' (Ball et al., 2019, 1).

> Mercians, Granadines, Andalusians, Estremenians, Portuguese, Galicians, Asturians, Cantabrians, Basques, Navarrese, Aragonese, and of the kingdom of Castile. Who is unable to see and know how they differ from one another, not only in their countenance and in the features of their bodies, but also in the virtues and vices of the soul?[5]

Huarte maintained that, although originally shaped by environmental factors and still susceptible to changes in one's diet, these qualities could be retained by members of a given *nación* for long periods of time even if they were to change their location, citing Romani people as a salient example: 'for although over 200 years have passed since the first Gypsies came from Egypt to Spain, their descendants have not lost their delicate wit and cunning brought by their parents from Egypt, nor their toasted colour'.[6] With Europeans then actively expanding their reach over the globe through settlement as a means of securing and enforcing initial claims of discovery and possession, the idea of a transportable yet stable body held some reassurances.

European medicine had long turned its eye to non-normative bodies, constructing them as such precisely by describing and emphasising their perceived exceptionality, such as in the case of the Jew, the African and the Moor. Pejorative assessments on Blackness have an extensive history in the European imagination. Far from being an American phenomenon, as James H. Sweet argued decades ago, the history of racialised discourse in the Iberian Peninsula dates back to at least the eighth century and draws upon Islamic practices for distinguishing between white, light-skinned and sub-Saharan African enslaved people, views that in turn impacted the ideology of later Western racial imagery. Sweet traced such distinctions through period terminology and showed how 'over time, Iberian Christians became acquainted with the Muslim system of Black slavery and adopted the same sets of symbols and myths, with additional arguments. Not only were Blacks non-Christians, but they were the Muslims' servants, the heathen's heathen' (1997, 149). He cites the example of an eleventh-century scholar writing in Toledo, Said al-Andalusi, who described 'the blacks, who live at the extremity of the land of Ethiops, the Nubians, the Zanj and the like' as having temperaments that

5 'Y vese claramente por experiencia cuánto disten los griegos de los escitas, y los franceses de los españoles, y los indios de los alemanes, y los de Etiopía de los ingleses. Y no solamente se echa de ver en regiones tan apartadas; pero si consideramos las provincias que rodean a toda España, podemos repartir las virtudes y vicios, … consideremos el ingenio y costumbres de los catalanes, valencianos, murcianos, granadinos, andaluces, extremeños, portugueses, gallegos, asturianos, montañeses, vizcaínos, navarros, aragoneses, y los del riñón de Castilla. ¿Quién no ve y conoce lo que estos difieren entre sí, no sólo en la figura del rostro y la compostura del cuerpo, pero también en las virtudes y vicios del ánima?' (1989, 247).

6 'con haber más de doscientos [años] que vinieron de Egipto a España los primeros gitanos, no han podido perder sus descendientes la delicadeza de ingenio y solercia que sacaron sus padres de Egipto, ni el color tostado' (1989, 523).

'become hot and their humours fiery, their colour black and their hair woolly. Thus, they lack self-control and steadiness of mind and are overcome by fickleness, foolishness and ignorance' (1997, 146). Geraldine Heng explains how this process that 'anatomize[d] alien nations, populations and races' then turned inward 'secur[ing] and stabiliz[ing] the moorings of what it meant to be Christian and European' (2007, 262). Humoral medicine certainly assisted in accommodating a phenomenological experience of perceived racial difference. But anatomy, given the ways in which it would develop and expand as a field of enquiry in the sixteenth century, would prove a less reliable ally epistemologically.

Although the *Examen* tends to be thought of as unusual in that it broached the subject of physiological difference linked to ethnicity so strongly and directly relative to other texts of its time, it is wise to remember Huarte's trajectory, his education and profession, conditions that enabled him to arrive at the model he proposed and to formulate his views along the lines he did. He was not an outlier when it came to his training; he was a doctor with a degree in medicine from the University of Alcala who studied with distinguished medical authorities of the day like Fernando de Mena, Francisco Vallés and Cristóbal de Vega (Virués Ortega, Buela-Casal and Carpintero Capell, 2006, 234). Professionally, despite gaps in the archive, more recent appraisals of documentary evidence correct earlier misconceptions, indicating he enjoyed several years of active practice as a physician, earning him a reputation that led to an offer to teach medicine at university level (Virués Ortega, Buela-Casal and Carpintero Capell, 2006, 234–35). The *Examen* may have been innovative in making more explicit the connections between views on science and political theory in a comparative evaluation of the limits of human difference, but its author was not on the fringe of period medical thought. Likewise, we should also recall that several rising medical authors of the time would be based in Iberian cities that arguably reflected demographically the textual diversity Huarte conjured up on the page. Monardes's Seville, for instance, had experienced unprecedented growth in the sixteenth century, its population increasing from 55,000 in 1535 to 120,519 by 1585 (Ven Deusen, 2015, 235). As Nancy E. van Deusen notes, Seville 'was truly international, filled with diverse northern (Berber) and West African, Flemish, Portuguese, French, German, Basque, and Genoese' gathering also 'thousands of slaves from different parts of the world' which amounted to 6,327 by 1565, 'most of whom came from the sub-Saharan African territories of Guinea, Mina, Cabo Verde, and Angola' (Van Deusen, 2015, 9–10). While Spaniards continued to represent the overwhelming majority of inhabitants, the city's ethnic heterogeneity by the second half of the sixteenth century even elicited hyperbolic negative critiques betraying xenophobic anxieties, such as that of an Italian ambassador who derisively compared Seville to a chessboard in its ratio of 'whites' to 'blacks' (Cavillac, 1992, 118).

And yet, despite numbers that paint a portrait of early modern European cities linked to trade as cosmopolitan places well accustomed to difference, a consideration of racial and ethnic minorities was not front and centre in medical thought or in medical practice, at least, not as it relates to the authors of Latin and vernacular medical sources. But the everyday demographic make-up of early colonial Mexico in the sixteenth century, with its disproportionately small number of Europeans, raises questions on how the medical literature of New Spain conceived of the variability of the human body, and the extent to which its ideas would have been on the same page as a text like the *Examen*. If a 1570 census of Mexico City counted only 8,000 Spanish males, compared to 60,000 Nahuas, 8,000 Africans, 2,000 *mestizos* and 1,000 *mulatos*, what was then the relationship between the body under scrutiny in early colonial medical literature and the real bodies of the people inhabiting that space?[7] Are assessments advanced by New World practitioners different from those espoused during the same period in a place like Padua or Paris because they arose in settings where the presumed European body template found itself not only in the company of *other* bodies but vastly outnumbered? Are we to understand that medical knowledge generated in early colonial Mexico would have concerned only a subset of the total population, chiefly Spaniards and their descendants, or was this a type of medicine for all bodies (or for every-body)? These questions go largely unacknowledged by the authors of early colonial anatomical and medical books who did not pose them in those terms, and whose works did not pursue a direct dialogue with the *Examen*; but they do speak to them.[8] As I show in this chapter, from Benavides in 1567 to Hinojosos, to Farfán, to Cárdenas in 1591: every single one of these New World authors explicitly mentioned Indigenous and

7 These numbers are drawn from Bennett (2003, 22) and Martínez (2004, 500–01) but need to be read with caution, as not only are they approximate, but they may not reflect how populations understood their own racial identities. It is also unclear how subjects of mixed African and Indigenous ancestry would be accounted for in one or more of the proposed categories. Bennett further notes that beyond the capital alone, 'by the end of the sixteenth century [Africans and their descendants] collectively rivaled, if not outnumbered, Spaniards throughout New Spain' (2003, 22). This trend in differential growth extended to the seventeenth century, with 'the African population [continuing] to outpace Spanish residents' (Schwaller, 2016, 62).

8 Like Benavides's *Secretos* (see chapter 1), the *Examen* is also mentioned by Leonard in his work on the early book trade in Latin America, but in relation to Peru rather than Mexico. In one of the surviving archival sources found by Leonard dating from 1583 there appears a request for twenty-five copies of San Juan's book intended to be sold locally (1992, 351). Notwithstanding its inclusion in the 1581 Portuguese Inquisitorial index, and in the 1583 Spanish Inquisitorial index, the *Examen* was an editorial phenomenon at the time, printed 10 times before the physician's death in 1588, and 18 more before the century drew to a close (see Orella, 1996, 51). While more research is needed to trace the exact circulation of San Juan's book in early New Spain, given the level of development of the book trade and the printing press in Mexico as compared to Peru at this juncture, it is unlikely the medical authors of Mexico were entirely unfamiliar with their colleague's ideas.

either African or African-descended people in their respective medical texts, even if they afforded them varying degrees of attention. The transplanting of European anatomical and physiological tenets into the social fabric of New Spain, captured in the literary representation of that exercise, tested the limits of a normative notion on the body well before cognate debates surfaced in Western scientific circles, turning early colonial discourse into a site where emerging ideas on racial difference were alternately contested and reaffirmed.[9]

The first pages of Alonso López de Hinojosos's *Svmma, y recopilacion de chirvgia, con vn Arte para sangrar muy vtil y prouechosa* (1578)[10] [Surgical compendium with a very useful and profitable art for bloodletting] counted on the support of three very distinguished readers in the context of New World medical practice. Juan de la Fuente, the first professor to teach medicine at the University of Mexico, vouched for the ample experience of its author, whom he knew to have practised 'the art of surgery' for many years, not just in Mexico but also during his younger days back in Spain (1977, 74). Agustín Farfán (whose biography will be discussed more fully in chapter 3), hard at work at the time finishing his own manuscript on anatomy and surgery, confessed that, because of this very task, he had not been able to assist as much as he would have liked to in the correction of the *Svmma*. Nonetheless, he claimed to have read Hinojosos's effort cover to cover, deeming it very useful 'for the land in which we find ourselves', and thought highly of its author, whom he described as an inquisitive, experienced and 'good Christian man' (1977, 72). Last, but not least, the more careful endorsement and revision of the text came from Francisco Bravo, by then the author of the first medical book printed in the New World,[11] who added that the *Svmma* would be of special interest to those who lived in the more remote areas of New Spain, in the fields and the mines, far from the resources that city dwellers enjoyed; readers who likely would not have had access to Bravo's own writings in Latin, nor the linguistic competence to have made sense of them (1977, 73). The man at the centre of these three converging opinions, however, was not a university-trained, accredited doctor as they were, but rather a surgeon and long-time nurse practitioner who would end his days modestly as a steward and gatekeeper at the Society of Jesus's Colegio Máximo. Yet with the *Svmma*, Alonso López

9 For an in-depth study on the medicalisation and pathologisation of racial categories linked to Africans and African-descended peoples in the context of the late eighteenth- and nineteenth-century Anglo Caribbean and the US South, see Hogarth (2017).

10 The page numbers in the quotations from the 1578 first printing of the text correspond to the modern edition of this version published by the Mexican Academia Nacional de Medicina in 1977, whereas the images are taken from the only known surviving copy held at the Huntington Library. Quotations and images from the 1595 edition are taken from an original copy at the John Carter Brown Library, one of the two known to still exist (the other one being housed at the British Library).

11 Bravo's text is the *Opera medicinalia, in q[ui]bus q[u]a[m] plurima extant scitu medico necessaria*, printed in 1570 in Mexico City by Pedro Ocharte.

de Hinojosos was to become the first author to publish a medical book written in a European vernacular language in the Americas.

Hinojosos was born around 1535 in Cuenca, Spain, and possibly trained as a barber and *cirujano romancista* [romance surgeon] but received no formal education. He lived in Seville in the late 1550s and early 1560s, likely the city where he met Fuente. On his arrival in Mexico, which occurred at some point before 1567, he worked first at the Hospital de la Concepción de Nuestra Señora that had been founded by Hernán Cortés, and later at the Hospital Real de los Naturales where he remained for the next 14 years.[12] His text would be published a second time before the seventeenth century, in a much-expanded edition that appeared in 1595 as the *Svmma y recopilacion de cirvgia, con vn arte para sangrar, y examen de barberos* [Surgical compendium with an art for bloodletting and an exam for barbers]. The two versions of the *Svmma* are quite different, with the second almost doubling the first in length, and making a series of changes, particularly in regards to its use of Indigenous herbal remedies as well as with the inclusion of sections on women's medicine and childbirth (topics discussed in greater detail in chapter 3).

Historians have tended to dismiss the level of innovation of the *Svmma* as a scientific project on the grounds that it relied heavily on older sources such as Aristotle, Guy de Chauliac and Juan de Vigo.[13] Its watershed status as a work written in Spanish rather than Latin is noted, and Hinojosos's role in conducting dissections is usually acknowledged in passing, linked to Francisco Hernández, a key Spanish physician of the early modern period appointed by Philip II as New Spain's *protomédico* [chief medical officer] and whom Hinojosos assisted briefly (see chapter 4 for a fuller discussion of Hernández and his significance in the context of New World *materia medica*). But historians of medicine find little else to say about the *Svmma*'s contributions to medical practice. Although 'one of the most beautiful jewels of Mexican medical literature in the sixteenth century' (1980a, 168), wrote Germán Somolinos d'Ardois, 'were it not for the chapter devoted to sarsaparilla and a

12 For Hinojosos's biography, see Somolinos d'Ardois (1977) and López Piñero and López-Terrada (1992). Somolinos mentions Hinojosos came to Mexico accompanied by a wife and daughter, and remarried after her death going on to have two sons. After losing his second wife, he joined the Society of Jesus in 1585 and died in 1597. For a discussion on the relationship between hospitals and colonial governance in Mexico after Charles V's 1541 decree ordering that hospitals 'be founded in all Spanish and Indian towns', see Risse (2000, 67), and more generally Rodríguez-Sala (2005a and 2005b), as well as Muriel (1990). According to Rodríguez-Sala, a total of 33 hospitals were established in New Spain between 1521 and 1595, eight of them in Mexico City (2005a, 49).

13 See Somolinos d'Ardois (1980a, 1980b and 1977) and Skaarup (2015). López Piñero and López-Terrada buck this trend, however, by stressing that 'it is meaningless to compare the two versions of his book with the more innovative tendencies of European medicine of the time, as some commentators have done' given 'the objectives and educational background' of the author (1992, 180).

few sparse allusions in the rest of the text, it could have been written in any learned European setting of the time' (Somolinos d'Ardois, 1977, 4). Hinojosos was not too interested initially in the 'newly discovered' local medicinal plants, as Monardes and others would be, nor was he particularly keen on challenging claims by European authorities of the period.[14] The *Svmma* thus tends to get lost in the bigger picture, deprived of the lustre of the projects surrounding it.

But there is more to Somolinos's assertion than meets the eye. Indeed, Hinojosos *did not* write the *Svmma* in Europe where his book could have been yet one more surgical compendium that summarised ideas better expressed elsewhere; it probably would not have been written by someone like him at all, the task possibly falling on others much better positioned in relation to established academic circles. Bravo's backhanded praise, placing the relevance of the *Svmma* just outside the doors of Mexico City, despite the predominately urban experiences described in the book or its author's decidedly urban professional background, help us imagine a much less direct route for Hinojosos to have become a published author had he remained in Spain, let alone of a book that merited a second edition. A more productive reading of the *Svmma* emerges if we see it as a text composed from the distinct vantage point of a practitioner then participating in the consolidation of what would become one of the major colonial Spanish cities in the Americas, and under circumstances that require careful consideration. There is, for example, his initial lengthy exposition on the environment's effects on human temperaments:

> In March, April and May, which is spring, the body is ruled by blood. In June, July and August, which is summer, it is ruled by yellow bile. In September, October and November, which is the autumn, black bile rules, and in December, January and February, which is the winter, phlegm rules. And likewise, in a natural day of twenty four hours these four humours rule the human body, for from three in the morning to nine in the day, blood rules. And from nine in the morning until three in the afternoon rules yellow bile. And from three in the afternoon until nine in the evening rules black bile. And from nine in the evening until three in the morning phlegm rules. And thus we see competent doctors ascertain at what times the patient's malady or fever increases or decreases, to better judge the illness and know the humour that causes it.[15]

14 Hinojosos's mentions of Indigenous medicine increase from the first to the second edition and, in fact, he does engage in a strong but veiled attack on Monardes, one of the most respected medical sources of the day, in the 1595 version of the *Svmma*, as will be discussed in chapter 4.

15 'En marzo, abril y mayo, que es el verano, reina en el cuerpo humano la sangre. En junio, julio y agosto, que es el estío, reina la cólera. En septiembre, octubre y noviembre, que es el otoño, reina la melancolía y en diciembre, enero y febrero, que es el invierno, reina la flema. Y así mismo en el día natural de veinticuatro horas reinan en el cuerpo humano estos cuatro humores, porque desde las tres de la mañana hasta

That this would be so in the Cantabrian mountains or off the coast of Naples would surprise no educated person of the time who had a basic familiarity with natural history. Yet, the notion that these same regular and predictable processes were occurring all along the Torrid Zone runs quietly counter to expectation. The influential Jesuit scholar and theologian José de Acosta would still find it necessary to explain to the readers of his *Historia natural y moral de las Indias* [*Natural and moral history of the Indies*] (1590) that New Spain and Peru were 'habitable and very abundantly inhabited, even though the ancients said it was impossible' (2002, 37). Acosta insisted on the error of older sources having judged the area 'completely uninhabitable owing to the excessive heat and proximity to the sun [that deprived it of] water and vegetation', when in fact, he stressed, 'all of this is the reverse' (2002, 37). The lack of difference is arguably the point in the *Svmma*, which presented Mexico as an extension of the expanding Spanish Empire, and as a natural setting where the embodied experiences of its recently arrived European inhabitants would be subject to equally foreseeable and controlled processes.

A mere *maestre*, in the context of the medical literature printed in Mexico during the early modern period, Hinojosos is the author who has to rely the most on personal experience and extra-academic education to carve out a position of epistemological authority, a feat he accomplished in no small part through his expertise in human dissection. Hinojosos appropriated the narrative model of the medieval surgical *exemplum* that had been used by figures such as Benavides (see chapter 1), retaining the elements of suspense and adventure, but expanding them beyond the living body so as to include also animated portrayals of dying and dead bodies whose insides go on to be represented through a poetics of disclosure and discovery. What in the *Secretos* had been narrative digressions, sometimes serving a comic effect, or vignettes that allowed European readers to peer into the mores of people living in strange and faraway places, become in the *Svmma* disciplined descriptions of case studies meant to highlight Hinojosos's ability to show the range of his practical knowledge, and to mark his level of privilege, even if relatively modest compared to that of fellow medical authors. Interspaced references to dissections throughout the text have the effect of imbuing the more formulaic or theoretical passages on humoral medicine or anatomical structures—chapters with titles such as 'What is a vein?' or 'What is an artery?'—with an experiential dimension confirmed by the surgeon's assumed sensorial contact with real bodies. One of the most important of these sections is found in the 1578 first edition on the subject of pestilence.

las nueve del día reina la sangre. Y desde las nueve de la mañana hasta las tres de la tarde reina la cólera. Y desde las tres de la tarde hasta las nueve de la noche reina la melancolía. Y desde las nueve de la noche hasta las tres de la mañana reina la flema. Y así veremos que los buenos médicos se informan a qué hora crece o mengua el accidente o calentura que tiene un enfermo para juzgar bien la enfermedad y de qué humor es causada' (1977, 97).

While not open to the general public, what would be remembered in later sources as the dissection of an 'Indian man' with cocoliste was a notorious event given its timing and context, which Hinojosos captures in full detail. Late in August 1576 he had been called to examine cocoliste victims by Mexican authorities who were right to fear the return of yet another massive wave of disease, one that would eventually result in the third major demographic dip among Indigenous populations of the region, claiming between 2 to 2.5 million lives by 1578. This grim chapter in New World medical history is considered to be of lesser consequence only because it is dwarfed in comparison with the scale of the ones that came before. While estimates vary, the epidemic in the period leading to the fall of Tenochtitlan killed between 5 to 8 million people from 1519 to 1520. Once colonial rule had been established, the cocoliste epidemic that set in from 1545 to 1548 claimed between 5 to 15 million, numbers that, if seen in context, can rightfully be considered 'one of the worst demographic catastrophes in human history, approaching even the Black Death of Bubonic plague' that had so changed the face of Europe in the fourteenth century (Acuña-Soto et al., 2002, 360).

Medical historians have different opinions as to the true identity of cocoliste and have also suggested the possibility that the use of the term by Indigenous populations and colonial authorities may have conflated different pathogens under one rubric. According to Raquel Álvarez Peláez, the first and second epidemic waves in New Spain were likely smallpox, and the third typhus, which she ascertains by comparing how they were described in *relaciones*, particularly in the work of Juan Bautista Pomar (1993, 266–76). From an epidemiological standpoint, Rodolfo Acuña-Soto and his team propose that the 1545 and 1576 epidemics were haemorragic fevers rather than smallpox, measles or typhus noting that the high rates of infection among Indigenous populations were not necessarily the result of their immune systems being unaccustomed to foreign infectious agents but could be explained by 'the extreme climatic conditions of the time' as well as the 'poor living conditions and harsh treatment of the native people under the encomienda system' (2002, 360). They attempt a modern diagnosis of the patients' clinical presentation and of the illness' prognosis insofar as it is possible to extract relevant data from period sources like Hinojosos's, leading them to conclude that 'cocoliztli was not pulmonary and may not have been a hantavirus', with patients expressing symptoms that 'are not consistent with known European or African diseases present in Mexico during the 16th century' (Acuña-Soto et al., 2002, 361, 360). More recently a joint interdisciplinary study including scholars at the Max Plank Institute for the Science of Human History, the University of Tübingen, Harvard University, the University of Zurich, the INAH and the Smithsonian Conservation Biology Institute have suggested that at least the 1545 epidemic could have been caused by *Salmonella enterica* (Vågene et al., 2018).

Hinojosos's highlighting of the 1576 episode speaks both to the magnitude of the illnesses' devastation in New Spain and to the fact that it was a defining moment in his life and career, where he had had the chance to come into contact with the highest political, religious and medical authorities in the land, many of whom he mentions by name in the text. As part of the official effort to respond to the looming threat, viceroy don Martín Enríquez had ordered 'the governor and the *alcaldes* of the Indigenous people and a translator or *naguatato* in his service' to visit 'more than one hundred sick people in one day, and when His Excellency heard of this, he summoned all the doctors who had a say in this, to ascertain what illness this was'.[16] At first 'the astrologers said the cause was an alignment of certain stars'; the doctors disagreed and 'said it was pestilence' which 'seemed probable given that it was summer and it had not rained in many years and the weather had changed quickly from excessively cold to excessively hot'.[17] However, seeing that 'the remedies of such famous doctors and their opinions were not yielding results, Enríquez ordered dissections to be performed'.[18] These were carried out at the Hospital Real de los Naturales and were supervised by Francisco Hernández, although Hinojosos would be the one to actually carry them out: 'I myself with my own hands undertook them', he writes.[19] The experience leads him to compose a detailed account of the illness's prognosis that weaves in and out of the skin's surface, and fluctuates between describing living bodies and dead ones:

> the liver of the patients was very hard and showed cirrhosis, protruding in such a deformed way that it looked like a bull's liver, raising the ribs upwards toward the chest very deformedly, because with its size and tumour it caused monstrosity. Their lungs were blue and dry; their gall bladders were blistered and obstructed and very large; the black bile that

16 'y sabido por el muy excelente señor virrey de esta Nueva España don Martín Enríquez lo que pasaba acerca de esta enfermedad, y para satisfacerse de la verdad, envió al gobernador y alcaldes de los naturales y a un intérprete o naguatato, de su casa … visitamos en un día más de cien enfermos y de que su excelencia esto supo, hizo llamar a todos los médicos que en esto tenían parecer, para certificarse qué enfermedad era' (1977, 207).

17 'Los astrólogos dijeron que la causa era conjunción de ciertas estrellas. Los médicos decían que era pestilencia. Esto cuadró por ser tiempo de estío y no haber llovido muchos años había y por hacer excesivo frío y escesiva calor en poca distancia de tiempo' (1977, 207).

18 'Sabido por el muy excelente señor virrey que los remedios de tan famosos médicos y sus pareceres no aprovechaban, mandó que se hiciesen anatomías' (1977, 209).

19 'yo propio por mis manos las hice estando presente el doctor Francisco Hernández' (1977, 209). While the autopsy is sometimes discussed in later sources as a single incident and as an anecdote attributed alternatively to Francisco Hernández or Juan de la Fuente, as both were also called to assist in the authorities' efforts, the wording in the *Svmma* is clear. It was not one but many autopsies that were performed, and they were carried out by Hinojosos. This arrangement was not unusual in the context of academic dissections where the figure touching the cadaver would be the surgeon-barber while the doctor would supervise and direct the proceedings, a division of labour strongly criticised by Vesalius, as mentioned in the previous chapter.

was within them rotted and the bile outside could not enter. Because of this the patients would be rendered very yellow and jaundiced. The urine they passed had a deep hue, like a mix of red and white wine, and was thick and dense. The ones who urinated often were the ones who survived. All the blood we drew from September to October was scarcely liquid, more like solid matter. Those afflicted by this illness had excessive thirst. They could not get enough water as the heat from the venom that they had in their stomachs and hearts was such, that these vapours would rise to the brain, so that within two days they would go mad, and we could not keep them lying down.[20]

The severity of the illnesses is conveyed by the degree to which both bodily functions and anatomical structures fail to conform to a normal, healthy, living template of the body, which is Hinojosos's main subject in his book, not disease. Recounting the cocoliste event served to underscore his experiential range, highlighting the access it had granted him to multiple cadavers, therefore justifying its inclusion in the overall economy of the project. But unsurprisingly, most of the allusions to human dissection in the *Svmma* refer to non-ailing bodies, namely injured patients or those of criminals, such as the passage the dissection of a man who had been quartered in Mexico, which he claimed had allowed him to confirm the correct placement of the liver (1595, fol. 85r).

The human digestive system in particular will be a key subject for Hinojosos, a conglomerate of structures he saw as linked to all the body's major functions. He warns against viewing problems in isolation: treating pain in the kidneys, or liver, or spleen, he argues, often fails to take into account the root causes that lead back to the gut: '[w]isdom dictates that he who has a healthy gut will have a good support for his bones. From which it follows that if there is no health in the gut, there will be no perfect health in the body'.[21] In a sequence

20 'tenían los enfermos el hígado acirrado y muy duro, que se les paraba tan deforme que parecía hígado de toro y alzaba las costillas hacia arriba y hacia el pecho muy deforme, porque con su grandeza y tumor hacía monstruosidad. Los bofes o livianos tenían azules y secos; la hiel apostemada y opilada y muy grande; la cólera que dentro estaba se pudría y la cólera que quedaba fuera no podía entrar dentro. Por esta causa se paraban los heridos de este mal muy amarillos y atiriciados. La orina que echaban los enfermos, era muy retinta como vino aloque y la orina muy gruesa y espesa. Los que orinaban mucho eran los que vivían. Cuanta sangre sacamos por sangrías en septiembre y octubre no tuvo ninguna acuosidad, sino era un témpano de materia. Los enfermos de esta enfermedad tenían excesiva sed. Nunca se hartaban de agua, porque era tanto el calor del veneno que en estómago y corazón tenían, que les subían aquellos humos al cerebro, que a dos días se tornaban locos, sin poderlos tener en la cama' (1977, 209–10).

21 'Y así lo dice la sabiduría, el que tuviere salud en su vientre, tendrá buen refresco para sus huesos. De do se sigue que si no hay salud en el vientre, no habrá perfecta salud en el cuerpo' (1595, fol. 125v).

of events resembling rumination in herbivorous mammals, according to the *Svmma*, ingested food does not all fit in the human stomach so a portion has to travel through the small intestines ['intestinos delgados'] into the cecum ['tripa ciega' or 'monóculo'], whence it returns to the stomach to finish being digested. Thanks to the opportunity made possible by a patient whose injury was so severe that it enabled Hinojosos to peer into the inner body, he is able to connect some of his observations on anatomy with his ideas on human physiology: 'I cured a man who was stabbed through the belly button tearing his cecum, from which a certain quantity of figs he had just eaten came out', which he saw as proof that undigested food could bypass the stomach to later return to it.[22] Hinojosos's interest lay in outlining a canonical idea of the body based not on repeated textual confirmation but on replicated experience, thus his insistent qualification when describing a particular event or dissection that he had, in fact, carried out 'many dissections' and had observed the phenomena being described 'many times' (1595, 85r). Hinojosos even proposed what in later centuries would be akin to a medical hypothesis, subjecting a living but soon-to-be-dead human specimen to a controlled experiment. In anticipation of gaining access to a condemned man's cadaver, 'and to certify even more this fact [that surplus undigested food was held in the cecum] I fed a man about to be quartered a certain quantity of fruit, and I found more than half of what he had eaten in the cecum, from which follows that it is true that both it and the stomach swell with food'.[23] The text is silent on how the postmortem examination came about, under whose authority, or whether it would have been atypical for a medical practitioner to be present both before and after an execution, granting him such a high level of participation and access. It also declines to elaborate on the subject's conceivable, although improbable, consent to being dissected postmortem.

Hinojosos's understanding of how intestinal functions transpire clearly differs not only from present-day ideas on human physiology but also did not match most other period sources; being 'unable to find it written' is what prompts his own decision to put pen to paper, he claims (1595, fol. 85v). In so doing he joined a long line of early modern medical practitioners and scientists who would come to both correct and incorrect conclusions in

22 'yo curé un hombre que le dieron una herida por el ombligo y le rompieron la tripa ciega, y por ella le salieron cierta cantidad de higos que acababa de comer' (1595, fol. 119r).

23 'por certificarme más desta verdad, queriendo llevar a hacer cuartos, un hombre le di a comer cierta cantidad de fruta, y hallé más de la mitad de lo que había comido en la tripa ciega, de donde se sigue ser verdad que se hinche de la comida a la par con el estómago' (1595, fol. 119r). This passage is as close as Hinojosos will come to discussing the issue of human vivisection, although it is a subject that arises in other period surgical texts in Spain, as in Juan Fragoso's *Cirvgia vniversal* [Universal surgery] (1581); Fragoso acknowledged its usefulness for ancient physicians but rejected it as barbarous. See chapter 3 for a fuller discussion of this source.

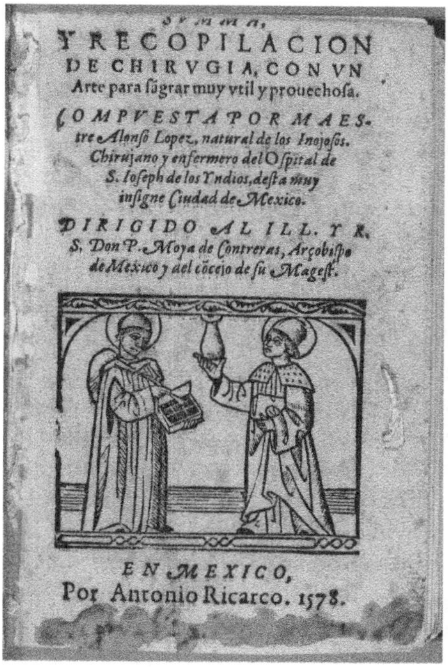

Y RECOPILACION
DE CHIRVGIA, CON VN
Arte para sãgrar muy vtil y prouechosa.
COMPVESTA POR MAES-
tre Alonso Lopez, natural de los Inojosos.
Chirujano y enfermero del Ospital de
S. Joseph de los Yndios, desta muy
insigne Ciudad de Mexico.
DIRIGIDO AL ILL. Y R.
S. Don P. Moya de Contreras, Arçobispo
de Mexico y del cõcejo de su Mageſt.
EN MEXICO,
Por Antonio Ricarco. 1578.

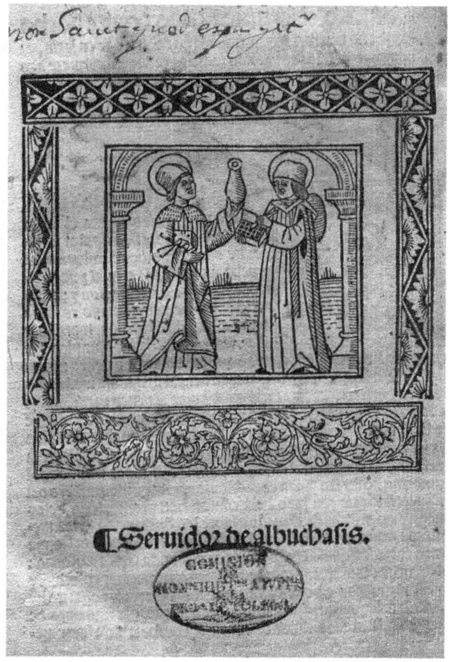

Seruidor de albuchasis.

Figures 2.1a and 2.1b. Title page of the first edition of Alonso López de Hinojosos's *Svmma, y recopilacion de chirvgia* [Surgical compendium] (1578) depicting the saints Cosmas and Damian (left), and title page of Alonso Rodríguez de Tudela's 1516 translation of tenth-century Andalusian physician Abū al-Qāsim Khalaf ibn ʿAbbās al-Zahrāwī, printed under the title of *Servidor de Albuchasis* [Albucasis's Servant] (right). The placement of the elements is reversed in the *Svmma*'s image, with the figure on the right holding the urine flask and the one on the left carrying the medicine box, supporting the idea that it is based on an earlier European template. Courtesy of the Huntington Library, San Marino, California (Item 106402), and the Biblioteca de Castilla-La Mancha, Borbón-Lorenzana Collection, Toledo respectively.

their interpretations of evidence, from Copernicus to Vesalius to figures of considerably lesser fame, like him. But he shared with them a similar epistemological view that increasingly sought and valued the accumulation of experiential data even if that process led to a challenge of earlier models or demanded the creation of new ones.

The shift in visual imagery from the first edition of the *Svmma* to the second attests to the increasing influence of this evolving mindset. The first printing had included three images: a woodcut of Saint John the Baptist, another of the Immaculate Conception and a title page showing Cosmas and Damian, who were the patron saints of physicians and surgeons (see figure 2.1a). In the image of the pair, the man on the left holds a medicine box and a spoon, while the one on the right balances a urine flask on his hand, which was a device used to determine a patient's humoral constitution by studying the liquid's colour. Cosmas and Damian were Christian martyrs from the third century who were said to have practised medicine free of charge and who, according to legend, had miraculously performed a successful homoplastic limb transplant, grafting the leg of an Æthiopian man onto the body of a non-Black patient. Representations of the pair carrying out the famed surgical procedure, or standing alongside one another holding objects related to medicine, were common in medieval European iconography.[24] In the case of Hinojosos's text, the formal elements in the *Svmma*'s image link it to Alonso Rodríguez de Tudela's translation of Abū al-Qāsim Khalaf ibn ʿAbbās al-Zahrāwī, the tenth-century physician whose text had been published in Valladolid in 1516 as the *Servidor de Albucasis* [Albucasis's Servant] (see figure 2.1b). As was often the case when a printer wanted to reproduce a design from another text but did not own the wood blocks that had been used to create it, an artist would be commissioned to draw a new image closely based on the original from which another block was carved, a process that resulted in a similar, but inverted print. While it has not been possible to ascertain whether the image on Hinojosos's first edition was commissioned locally or made previously in Europe and then brought to Mexico, the link to Tudela's text at some point in its history is fairly certain given the duplication of formal elements, such as the ermine coat in one of the men, and the folds in the cloth of the gowns.[25]

However, the second printing of the *Svmma* removes the allegorical images of the saints altogether. The woodcut in the title page harkening back to older medical practices is replaced by the emblem of the Society of Jesus, a seal present in several other Mexican imprints during the century's final decade and which associated Hinojosos's text to new projects that differed in language and subject matter but that shared a common link to the Order (see figure 2.2). Perhaps more suggestively, the second edition features an anatomical

24 On the importance of depictions of Cosmas and Damian in medieval and early modern European culture, and in particular on how sixteenth-century Castilian depictions of this legend informed 'the iconography of the enslaved Afro-Hispanic subject', see Fracchia (2019, 121–53).

25 Further research on early modern visual culture could reveal whether the two images share a common template, or whether other versions of the design exist that could have mediated the duplication of visual elements. For example, the image on the title page of Mondino de Liuzzi (1270–1326) *Mundinus de Anathomia* (Salamanca, 1540) also resembles very closely the one in the *Servidor*, duplicating gestures and angles, but is unlikely to be a bridge to the *Svmma* as it suppresses elements like the ermine coat. The title page of the 1524 Spanish edition of the *Thesaurus pauperum* [Medical book known as the treasure of the poor] written by Arnau de Vilanova (1238?–1311) features a design that also seems to go back to the *Servidor's* image given its placement of elements, although with more substantial alterations and greater artistic licence.

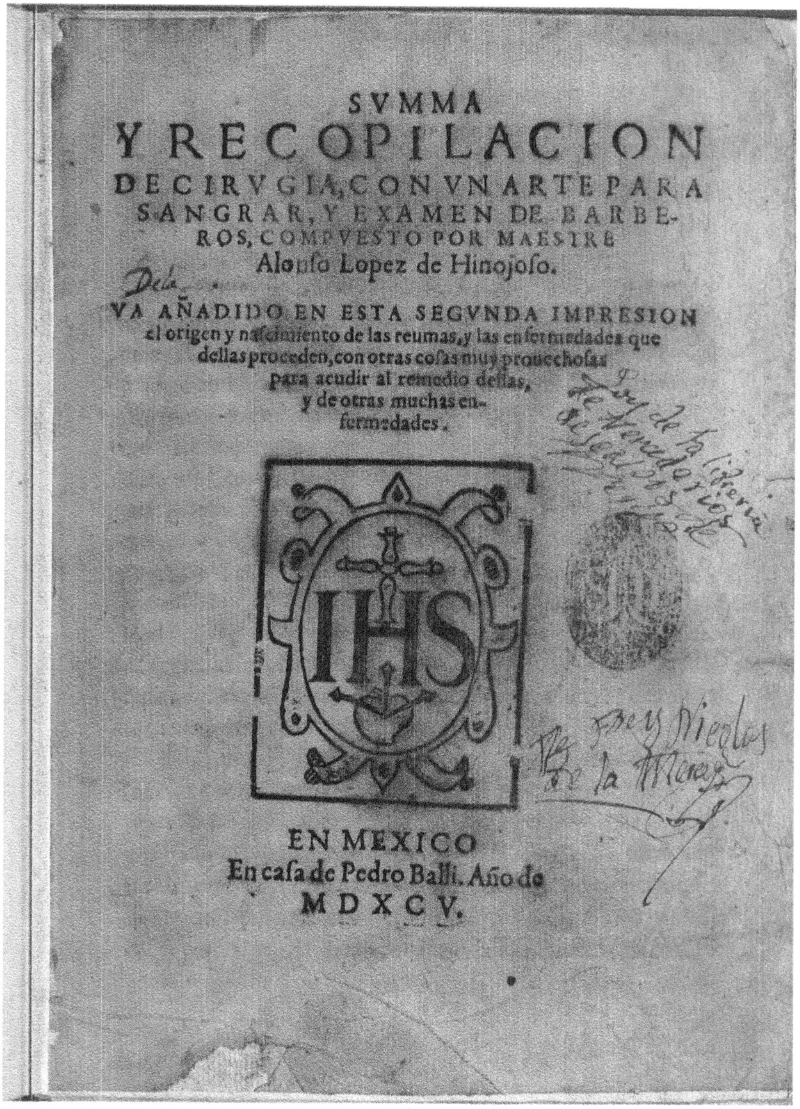

SVMMA
Y RECOPILACION
DE CIRVGIA, CON VN ARTE PARA
SANGRAR, Y EXAMEN DE BARBE-
ROS, COMPVESTO POR MAESTRE
Alonſo Lopez de Hinojoſo.

VA AÑADIDO EN ESTA SEGVNDA IMPRESION
el origen y naſcimiento de las reumas, y las enfermedades que
dellas proceden, con otras coſas muy prouechoſas
para acudir al remedio dellas,
y de otras muchas en-
fermedades.

EN MEXICO
En caſa de Pedro Balli. Año de
MDXCV.

Figure 2.2. Title page of Alonso López de Hinojosos's second edition of the *Svmma* (1595), where the religious image of the first printing is replaced with the emblem of the Society of Jesus. This specific woodcut design had been used by Balli before in Fray San Juan Buenaventura's *Mistica Theologica* (1594), and would be used again in Manuel Alvares's *Emmanvelis Alvarie* (1595) and Antonio del Rincón's *Arte Mexicana* (1595). The repeated use of the emblem in projects that differed in language and subject matter visually underscored for the readers of New Spain Jesuit claims of a superior and wideranging intellectual reach. Courtesy of the John Carter Brown Library.

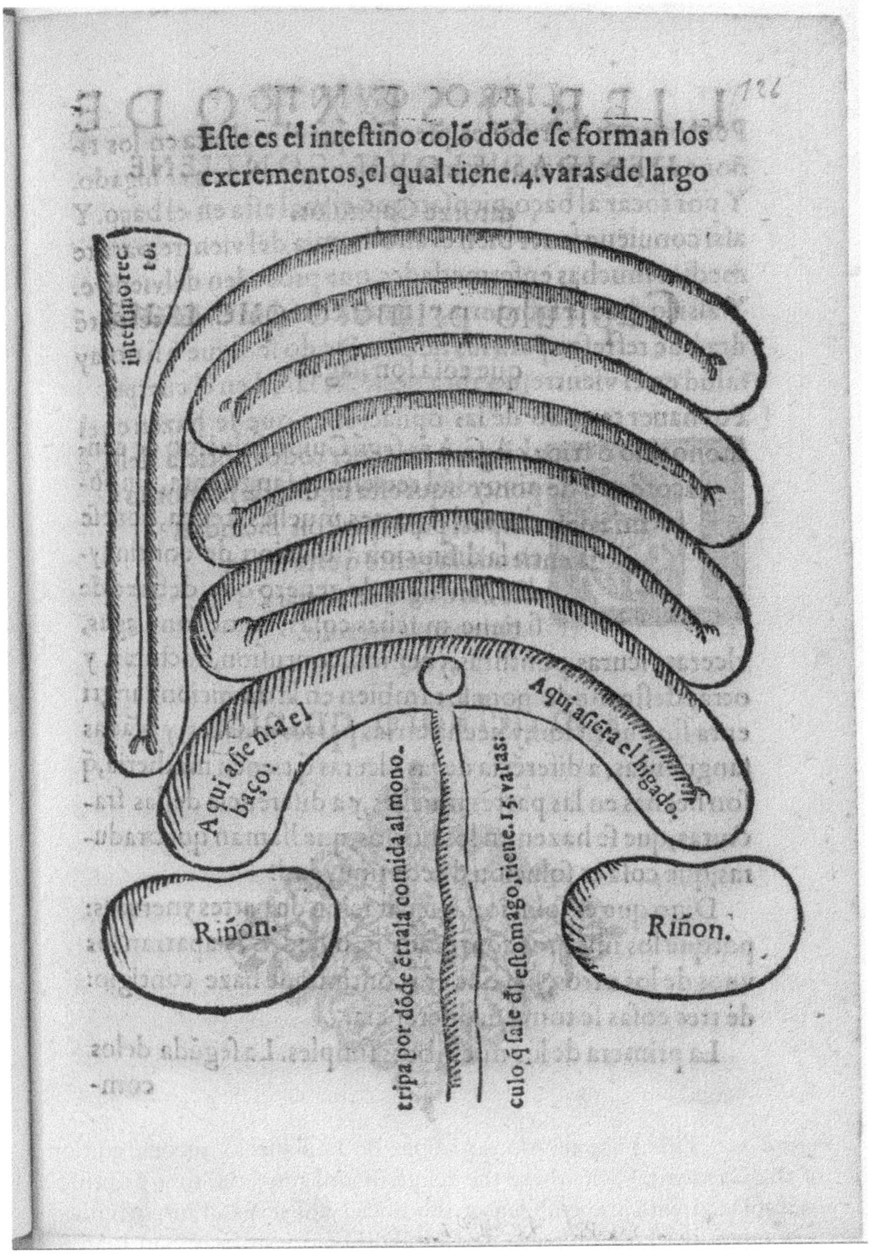

Figure 2.3. Folio 126r of Alonso López de Hinojosos's second edition of the *Svmma* (1595), showing the intestines flanked by the kidneys. The anatomical image is upside down, with a portion of the small intestine visible bottom centre, and the rectum placed on the top left side. Courtesy of the John Carter Brown Library.

image, a diagram of the gut flanked by the kidneys (see figure 2.3), the second large anatomical illustration to be printed in the Americas.[26] The diagram is a combination of image and text, with labels placed directly on top or alongside the structures described. It shows a partial view of the small intestine (which is mostly off-scene) measuring 15 *varas*,[27] leading into the first part of the large intestine (alternatively referred to by Hinojosos as the *monóculo*, *tripa ciega*, or the *intestino colon*), measuring 4 *varas*, and connecting to the rectum [*intestino recto*]. Readers encounter the image upside down, as if standing behind a cadaver's head looking down at a body placed horizontally: 'here would lie the spleen' reads the text on the left (rather than the right), with a similar statement made about the liver on the opposite side of the page. Hinojosos's justification for including the diagram reads thus:

> Having just discussed the obstructions of the humours that occur in the *monóculo* or *tripa ciega*, and because not all have news of it, I have decided to place here this figure on the anatomy of the gut, so that the people who live outside this city, who are the ones for whom I write, may easily understand it.[28]

Anatomical images were not at all common in books printed in New Spain, even for city-dwellers, either in the sixteenth century, or indeed in the following one, as the level of technological sophistication in engraving methods achieved by print shops operating in major cities across Europe would not transfer to the New World until centuries later. Prior to Hinojosos's diagram of the gut there had only been one other locally printed anatomical image of comparable size, found in Bravo's *Opera medicinalia*, an illustration of the subclavian vein joining the superior vena cava, which had been modelled on an earlier diagram from Vesalius's *Venesection epistle*.[29]

In the context of medieval and early modern medical illustrations, the innovation of the image in the 1595 *Svmma* lies in its semantic tension as both a counterfeit and an indexical diagram. Counterfeits, as Sachiko Kusukawa explains, 'claimed to convey the truth of a particular person or event from which the viewer was separated in space and/or time' (2012, 9). In surgical

26 The first edition of Farfán's *Tractado* (1579) included small medical illustrations, including one of an anatomical structure. See Pérez Marín (2020, 105–06).

27 According to the work of Brading, *varas* or 'Castilian yards', were equivalent to '33 English inches or 0.835 metres' (2008, xiv).

28 'Por haber tratado de las opilaciones que se hacen en el monóculo o tripa ciega, y no tener todos noticia de ella, he acordado de poner aquí esta figura de la anatomía de las tripas, para que con facilidad la entiendan la gente que está fuera de esta ciudad que es para quien yo la escribo' (1595, fol. 125v).

29 The image, which offers an incorrect appraisal of the heart because it does not account for the left–right inversion resulting from the process of copying the original image, appeared in a section of the *Opera* where Bravo turned to Vesalius in an effort to refute Monardes (see chapters 1 and 4).

literature, counterfeits could add 'vivid, particular details' which helped the reader 'feel as if they were firsthand (sic) witnesses to the event' (2012, 9). Their presence 'in printed books on surgery or medicinal plants … did not signal new developments in anatomical or botanical knowledge, nor did [they] necessarily reflect any new observational attitudes on their authors' (2012, 19). The indexical anatomical and botanical images that arose in the first half of the sixteenth century often deliberately eschewed the naturalism of the counterfeit, representing artistic examples that could never be found in nature. A single plant would be shown in different stages of growth and decay, all occurring simultaneously, or there could be an image that grafted onto a single structure different varieties of a plant's flowers in an effort to encompass all known variations. Likewise, anatomical images often turned to geometry, with structures shown schematically and outside the body, so as to try to endow an individual case with the universality and regularity of mathematics (Kusukawa, 2012, 193). However, in works such as his *De humani corporis fabrica* (1543), Vesalius recuperated elements of realism associated with counterfeits, like the shading of structures or the inclusion of backgrounds, placing them in a dialogue with the indexical impetus of the anatomical diagram. The interaction was negotiated through a new aesthetics that added a layer of anthropomorphic unreality, as evidenced by numerous skeletons and flayed bodies displayed in unlikely positions suggesting animation.[30]

In the case of the 1595 *Svmma*, no prior templates of the gut image shown in the text have surfaced thus far, although the possibility that it was based on an as yet unidentified source cannot be ruled out. While Vesalius was deeply involved in the creation of the images accompanying his work, a feature he often stressed to readers in his prose, the relationship between author, illustrator and engraver in other sixteenth-century anatomical print materials could be structured differently. A reliance on a prior model did not necessarily undermine an author's purchase over the information being presented. Such was the case, for example, of Charles Estienne's *De dissectione partium corpori humani libri tres* [On the dissection of the parts of the human body] (Paris 1545), along with Vesalius's *Fabrica*, considered a landmark text in the history of medicine for its use of early modern visual technology to discuss matters of anatomy. Estienne, in collaboration with fellow surgeon

30 Examples of 'living cadavers' used as anatomical illustrations are a mainstay in some of the more influential medical books of the sixteenth century, including not just the *Fabrica* but also Jacopo Berengario da Carpi's *Anatomia Carpi* (1535), Juan Valverde de Amusco's *Historia de la composición del cuerpo humano* [Anatomy of the Human Body] (1556) and Charles Estienne's *La dissection des parties du corps humain* [On the Dissection of the Parts of the Human Body] (1546). The preference for including these kinds of representations in anatomical literature would linger all the way to the eighteenth century to the point that their fictional charge is often overlooked because they become subsumed in a Western visual vocabulary.

Étienne de la Rivière, recycled woodcuts from non-anatomical sources for some of his illustrations, cutting away subsections within the larger image where more detailed diagrams were inserted, leaving a telltale line in the area where the change had taken place.[31] While the degree to which Hinojosos himself participated in the artistic rendition of the medical illustration in his book is not known, he expressed a clear ownership over the image, stressing its correspondence to his own written account of physiological processes and first-hand observations. His choice to use the illustration of body parts rather than the whole body, and of labels that highlighted a connection to the surrounding written text, link the second edition of the *Svmma* to the more modern approaches of contemporaries such as Vesalius and Juan Valverde de Amusco. And yet his explanation that the image is supplemental and for the unlearned reader, as well as the level of detail in the shading, with the light source clearly being on the right rather than the left, still connect it with the older tradition of the counterfeit, which claimed to represent a single specimen that had once existed or been observed. In this case, the tension is resolved in favour of the former rather than the latter through the use of language: the image is not a portrayal of an individual instance of a dissection, sharing the exact measurement of that particular specimen, but rather an indexical image of a canonical body, purporting to describe repeating phenomena and spatial arrangements in the third person. The image does not show the insides of *a* body, but rather of *the* body.

Whereas the demographic proportion that marked Europeans as a very small minority is brought out in early colonial sources relating to the era of conquest and colonisation, and is also reflected in the number of bilingual and trilingual early Mexican imprints for proselytising, by the last third of the sixteenth century non-Spanish populations were increasingly rendered invisible in literary and artistic texts.[32] This phenomenon would only become more pronounced in the seventeenth century when, despite non-Spaniards comprising the overwhelming majority of the artisanal and labour workforces powering Mexico's cultural and artistic flourishing, a sense of regional colonial identity would remain firmly Europe-facing. The early medical texts of Mexico do more than just reflect this path: they

31 The woodcuts in this text are accessible via the National Library of Medicine's Historical Anatomies on the Web portal (https://www.nlm.nih.gov/exhibition/historicalanatomies/home.html).

32 See Stephanie Merrim's analysis of local literary representations of Mexico City during the last quarter of the sixteenth century, which builds on Francisco Cervantes de Salazar's earlier mid-century appraisal of the city as an ordered, European space tarnished by the presence of Indigenous people. In particular, see her discussion on Eugenio de Salazar y Alarcón's 'Bucólica' (written c.1597), which she describes as '[a]n operatic, sublime, imperialist extravaganza' that uses lyric to present readers with a view of that colonial space though 'fetishized, hypertrophic whiteness' (2010, 84, 87, 310).

help to chart it by articulating a shared Spanish-speaking platform with fellow European and European-descended readers, often referred to in the first person plural, set against a horizon of Indigenous peoples, Africans and African-descended groups, on the one hand, and, on the other, confronting what was seen as the threat of emerging physiological ideas on the transformative and degenerative power of a New World environment acting on European bodies.

Medical authors in Mexico were grappling with arguments that had begun to compare the New World unfavourably to the Old, threatening to taint assessments on the aptitudes and virtues of the sons and daughters of Spaniards being born outside Spain. The drive to create different, separate and stable bodily identities for Europeans sharing a common New World space with other *naciones* arises with a sense of urgency during the late sixteenth century in Juan de Cárdenas's *Primera parte de los problemas y secretos marauillosos de las Indias* [First part of the problems and marvellous secrets of the Indies], published in 1591.[33] Cárdenas was probably born in 1563 in Constantina, a town close to Seville, and sailed to the New World when he was around 14 years old. He studied at the Colegio Máximo, and later became part of the first cohort of doctors trained at the University of Mexico by Fuente. He would aspire to teach medicine himself at his alma mater after Fuente's death, but he was unable to secure the post immediately, twice losing out to competitors. He eventually succeeded in 1607 but only briefly, dying two years later. As Jorge Cañizares-Esguerra has convincingly argued, Cárdenas's book is worth noting because it offered a reasoned, scientific exposition on the intellectual superiority of the *criollo* vis-à-vis the peninsular-born Spaniard. Cárdenas believed that while those born in Spain were choleric, the Spaniards born in the New World developed a choleric-sanguine constitution, which made them weaker physically, but endowed them with a keener intellect.[34] 'Those born in the Indies are generally sanguine', he explains, 'which speaking according to Galen's doctrine means that they are of a hot and humid complexion.'[35] Yet because the 'Spanish *nación* is characteristically choleric', the sanguine constitution of children and youngsters was partially overcome in adulthood by the traits inherited from their parents. Like Huarte, Cárdenas accepts the notion of a biological transference of traits from parents to children, and does not differentiate between the contribution of the father versus the mother. He expresses the idea both through circumlocution with the verb 'to participate', in constructions such as 'the dryness of this yellow bile participated by the parents is tempered in the children' ['la nación española es de suyo colérica [y la]

33 See note 21 in the Introduction.

34 See Cañizares-Esguerra, 2006.

35 'los nacidos en Indias son generalmente sanguíneos, que hablando conforme a la doctrina de Galeno es decir que son de complexión caliente y húmeda' (1591, fol. 178v).

sequedad desta cólera participada de los padres, se templa en los hijos'] (1591, fol. 179r), as well as with the verb 'to inherit', when he refers to 'inherited diseases, by which I mean that they are inherited from parents and grandparents' ['males hereditarios, quiero decir que se heredan de padres y abuelos'] (1591, fol. 218v). It was a phenomenon that, according to Cárdenas, could be confirmed through personal experience:

> To show and give true testimony that all those born in the Indies are of sharp, superior and delicate intellect, let us compare one from here, with another recently arrived from Spain, and let this be the manner, that the one born in the Indies not be raised in one of these great and famous cities of the Indies, but in a poor and barbarous Indian village, only in the company of four farmers, and let the *cachupín*, or recently arrived man from Spain be from a village, and let the two interact so they may talk and converse with one another: we will hear the Spaniard born in the Indies, speak in such a polished, courtly and curious manner, with such ornament, and gentleness, and rhetorical style not learned or artificial, but natural, that he seems to have spent all his life at court and in the company of very learned and discreet people; on the contrary you will see the *chapetón*, unless he has been raised among city folk, that there is no tree with a coarser bark and as clumsy as he; for the demeanour of one is so different from the other, one so clumsy the other so lively, that that no man regardless of how ignorant, could not plainly see which one is the *cachupín* and which one was born in the Indies.[36]

What is striking in Cárdenas's exercise is how the description is couched in the language of empiricism, anticipating the idea of having a controlled variable in an experiment. The preconditions for both subjects should be equal to rule out other factors and prevent differences in upbringing from affecting the outcome. Second, the epistemological stability of the observation lies in the sum of others' experiences as witnesses, and not just his own

36 'Para dar muestra, y testimonio cierto, de que todos los nacidos en Indias sean a una mano de agudo trascendido y delicado ingenio, quiero que comparemos a uno de los de acá con otro recién venido de España, y sea ésta la manera, que el nacido en las Indias no sea criado en alguna destas grandes y famosas ciudades de las Indias, sino en una pobre y bárbara aldea de Indios, sólo en compañía de cuatro labradores, y sea asimismo el cachupín o recién venido de España criado en aldea, y júntense éstos que tengan plática y conversación el uno con el otro, oiremos al Español nacido en las Indias, hablar tan pulido cortesano y curioso, y con tantos preámbulos delicadeza, y estilo retórico, no enseñado ni artificial, sino natural, que parece que ha sido criado toda su vida en corte, y en compañía de gente muy hablada y discreta, al contrario verán al chapetón, como no se haya criado entre gente ciudadana, que no hay palo con corteza que más bronco y torpe sea, pues ver el modo de proceder en todo el uno tan differente del otro, uno tan torpe, y otro tan vivo, que no hay hombre, por ignorante que sea, que luego no eche de ver, cuál sea cachupín, y cuál nacido en Indias' (1591, fols. 176v–177r).

assessment. Behaviour, measured primarily through eloquence, becomes the external manifestation of a physiological process, one that is not immune to external factors, but that is stable enough phenomenologically to be systematically repeated and applicable to all those born in the Indies.

The passage's choice of nomenclature is more important than it would seem in light of another period text that also discussed the idea using similar language. Cárdenas refers to the children of Spaniards born in the Indies as 'españoles de Indias', taken to mean Spaniards 'of' or 'from' the Indies. Other times he avoids the demonym altogether, as in the passage just cited, 'those born in the Indies' [*los nacidos en Indias*] although he never uses the latter in a context where the reader would presume he could mean African-descended people or Indigenous people also born there. *Criollo*, however, is conspicuously absent.

Royal chronicler Juan López de Velasco's *Geografía y descripción universal de las Indias* [Geography and universal description of the Indies] (1574) was one of the first texts to use the word *criollo* in print in the sense that it would have during most of the colonial era, that is, to describe individuals who claimed to be descended from Spaniards and who denied or minimised any Black or Indigenous ancestry. In a section entitled 'Of the Spaniards born in the Indies' López de Velasco contended that:

> The Spaniards that go to those parts and live there for a long time, with the mutation of the skies and the temperaments of the regions are not immune to receiving some difference in the colour and *calidad* of their persons; but those who are born there, and are known as *criollos*, and are in everything taken and regarded as Spaniards, are already different in their colour and size … not only are their bodily qualities changed, but those of the soul follow the body, and are changed too.[37]

While López de Velasco positions his remarks as if he accepted the premise that Spaniards could be born in different places given the section's axiomatic heading, he in fact sets out to undermine that idea by clarifying it is a simile. Members of this other group are *like* Spaniards, 'taken and regarded' as if they were the same, but not by him necessarily and soon, not by his readers either once they finish reading his physiological explanation. Further, the use of the third person conveys the idea of collective support for his position and of a widespread use of *criollo*; it is not that he is proposing a new convenient disambiguation but rather reporting on its purported generalised use.

37 'Los españoles que pasan a aquellas partes y están en ellas mucho tiempo, con la mutación del cielo y del temperamento de las regiones aun no dejan de recibir alguna diferencia en el color y calidad de las personas; pero los que nacen de ellos, que llaman criollos, y en todo son tenidos y habidos por españoles, conocidamente salen ya diferenciados en el color y en el tamaño … y no solamente en las calidades corporales se muda, pero en las del ánimo suelen seguir las del cuerpo, y mudando él se alteran también' (1971, 19–20).

However, this term then had an active derogatory connotation. It was used during the same period in the Caribbean to mean enslaved Africans born in the New World, and closer to Cárdenas's geographic context, in Mexico City and Puebla, it could refer both to that group as well as to Mexican-born subjects of mixed African/Spanish ancestry into the next century.[38] These associations may explain Cárdenas's sustained exclusionary performance throughout the whole of his book. For López de Velasco, all Spaniards in the Indies were subject to being transformed if they spent too much time there, a change that was definitive if they were born outside Europe. As observed by the late José Juan Arrom, the idea of such a transformation was so contentious that, as early as 1576, the Council of the Indies ordered that the passage quoted earlier be suppressed from future printings of the *Geografía*.[39] By the time the *Problemas y secretos* was published in 1591, both writer and reader would have been aware that Cárdenas's insistence in opting for the verbose 'Spaniard of the Indies' in Book 3 was not accidental.

As Cañizares-Esguerra has explained:

> Creole colonists responded to disparaging European views of the climate and constellations of Spanish America as threatening and degenerating by suggesting that there were racially innate body types which changed only slightly under new environmental influences, thus rejecting long-held theories of temperaments and complexions according to which 'European' bodies became 'Indian' ones under the climate and stars of the New World. (2005, 427)

However, Cárdenas's own position at this historical juncture is not yet that clearly defined in regard to the stability of race. In his model, the bodily changes that came with the new setting were not slight but profound, and were creating a number of serious health issues to which the medical explanations in his book turn to over and over. The newer generations of Spaniards born in the Indies were not healthy: they died younger than their counterparts in Spain, and they did not live to old age as had their parents before them. Cárdenas takes pains to differentiate between 'muerte natural' [death by natural causes] and 'muerte violenta', which for him included illness (1591, fols. 172v–173v). In his model, the Spaniards of Mexico's intellectual acuity came at a cost, but measures could and should be taken to mitigate the pernicious effects of the land's excessive humidity and the poor quality of foods it was able to produce, two of the main reasons for the predicament, in his opinion (1591, fol. 174v, fol. 165v). That the *Problemas y secretos* provided concrete solutions for how to manage these health hazards effectively was one of the book's main justifications. A diet that avoided delicacies [*manjares*] and overindulgence, that understood how to combine local products effectively to bring out their beneficial properties and supress

38 See Martínez (2008, 160).

39 Cited in Zamora, note 17 (1988, 174).

or minimise harmful ones, as well as a more robust work ethic that did not fall prey to idleness [*ociosidad*], could combat the noxious effects of the land (1591, fols. 175v–176r).

Whereas centuries later important Mexican intellectuals would speak of Cárdenas as an ally of the *criollo* cause, there are parts of the *Problemas y secretos* that betray an adversarial stance between him and his contemporaries in New Spain (see chapter 4 for further discussion on this point). Notwithstanding the positive consequences Cárdenas adduces of being endowed with superior eloquence and enhanced intellectual abilities, there are signs that those he spoke of would not have welcomed the idea of a transformed body regardless; after all, 'Spaniards of the Indies' paradoxically reinforced the point that a distinction was appropriate, and even demonstrable. In fact, Cárdenas discloses that he is overriding *criollos*' objections by agreeing with the opinion that there was indeed a mutable Spanish body, giving us a rare glimpse of early colonial subjectivity and how members of that community would have felt about arguments that differentiated some of them from their Iberian kin. Spanish men born in New Spain do tend to die young, Cárdenas affirms patronisingly, even if there are those who 'think otherwise, mostly if they are born in this land, since they do not like to talk about this, they say that in this there is no difference, and that all the world is one'.[40] Even before Cervantes would have Sancho tell the same to Countess Trifaldi, opinionated colonists in Mexico are shown seeking refuge in the Spanish *Refranero* to push back against views that would make them different: 'todo el mundo es uno'.[41]

Cañizares-Esguerra is right to suggest that a racialised Spanish body would have been appealing to colonists, an idea worth supporting, institutionalising

40 'son de contrario parecer, mayormente si son naturales de esta tierra, como no gustan mucho de la plática, dicen que en esto no hay diferencia, y que todo el mundo es uno' (fol. 172r).

41 The phrase entered the repertoire of the early modern Spanish *Refranero* as a version of Petronius' 'Ubique medius caelus est'. Although there is no evidence Cárdenas had access to it, the phrase had also been used in writing in an American context by Tomás López Medel in his 'De los tres elementos, aire, agua y tierra' (unpublished in the sixteenth century), a treatise that according to Antonio Barrera-Osorio was 'the first attempt to present the nature of the New World within the classical categorization of the elements and their properties' (2006, 91). López Medel, however, had enlisted the phrase in a different context, to support the Lascasian view of Indigenous rationality: 'Of what I have stated above we can glean how true that other one's words were [Las Casas's]: that all the world is one, and that if the Indians deserved to be reprimanded for their mode of governance, we are far more deserving of censure given our abominable ways' (1990, 323). Cervantes, who made ample use of period popular sayings in the *Quijote*, most noticeably in the characterisation of his protagonist's squire, would have Sancho voice the sentiment in chapter 38 of the Second Part (1615): 'In Candaya too there are alguazils of the court, poets and roundelays, and so I swear that I imagine all the world is one' (1994, 846).

and policing, particularly to *criollos* as the colonial era wore on with successive waves of European immigration and increased miscegenation.[42] And throughout most of his book, Cárdenas stays within these lines by not making distinctions when narrating Spaniards' interactions with their environment, or even in sections where presumably being choleric versus choleric-sanguine could have made a difference to the effects of natural products being described. But voiced by someone who did not need to qualify his own *nación* (there is no redundant 'Spaniards of Spain' phrasing in the *Problemas y secretos*, nor any formulation akin to *peninsular*, a term already in use by 1555), his attempt to wrestle *criollo* away from voices like those of López de Velasco by conceding to a change but making a case that it could be for the better does not quite persuade. Despite his periphrastic rhetorical move bordering on *captatio benevolentiae* to circumvent terminology laden with controversy for local readers, his efforts may have fallen flat. While the *Problemas y secretos* would be read in the Americas in the seventeenth century (see chapter 4), his position in this regard may help to explain the book's underwhelming impact and relative obscurity in colonial letters going forward until its resurgence in the twentieth century.

In contrast, other parts of his argument reflected more closely emerging ideas on racial difference that would be developed in colonial thought going forward. These occur when he turns his attention instead to establishing the superiority of the Spanish body—no qualified demonyms then—by way of examples to non-European bodies using the tools of physiology. Activating some of the same language on Chichimecs found in sources like Gonzalo Fernández de Oviedo and José de Acosta, and noticeably heightening the dramatic weight of his prose through an uncharacteristic abundance of adjectives and the use of literary devices like pleonasm and metaphor, 'chichimecas' are described in resolutely negative terms:

> The Chichimeca nation are a barbarous and savage people, never conquered or controlled by any other *nación*. They are perpetually naked, live in rocky and uncomfortable areas, and their preference is to kill and take the lives not just of human kind but of any animal, large or small. They forgive no one, showing themselves to be cruel butchers. Tombs of human flesh are their stomachs, and this is their principal nourishment which, if lacking, they will substitute for raw animal meat, be it serpent, snake, toad, lizard; and if unavailable, turning then to roots or some wild fruits.[43]

42 For a consideration of how Hippocratic understandings of the body may have influenced later ideas on race in the context of castas and racially mixed populations, from the seventeenth to the nineteenth centuries, see López Beltrán (2007).

43 'La nación chichimeca es una gente bárbara salvaje jamás sujeta ni domada por otra nación alguna, tiene propiedad de andar perpetuamente desnuda, su habitación es entre fragosos riscos y peñascos, su propio oficio es matar y quitar vida no sólo al

Chichimecs' radical difference is confirmed by how their bodies respond to what are for Spanish bodies, positive and civilising changes to the environment:

> As brave, strong, sturdy and healthy as they are in their own lands, despite eating the worst nourishment, lack of sleep, and walking naked and barefoot, in coming under our power they are rendered miserable, weak and sickly despite access to comforts and being raised like people proper; he who would see a Chichimec hidden in the rocks looking like a devil later sees him amongst us turned into a weakling and the very picture of sickness and sorrow that no sooner has he felt the slightest little bit of pain or mildest bout of diarrhoea that he is immediately dead.[44]

The prose in this section continues to stand out from other parts of the *Problemas y secretos*, this time in its preference for diminutives used derisively to underscore contrasts. Mighty, undefeated and fearsome as they were prior to the arrival of Europeans, once 'under our power', not because of any mistreatment but as the natural result of being exposed to comforts and to being raised 'like people proper' [criándose como gente] they are unable to successfully adapt to change. Not unlike what he had argued in the description of Spaniards' transformation, there could be ways of mitigating negative effects, presumably maintaining their access to poor quality food, which 'for them it is healthy and very good',[45] or restoring the level of physical activity they had prior to entering an urban environment, being accustomed, as they were, according to Cárdenas, to 'running and jumping among the hills, where they release and consume with that strong exercise all their bad humours', hinting at an unsettling scientific basis for the benefits of hard labour, such as the mine work which figures like Cortés had deemed particularly apt for them specifically.[46] Almost a century after observers in Seville had judged the extremely high mortality rate of the Indigenous people who had been

género humano pero desde el menor hasta el mayor animal, y sabandija ninguno perdona, mostrándose enemiga cruel y carnicera a todo, son sus vientres sepultura de carne humana, y éste es su principal sustento y regalo, a cuya falta usan de carne cruda de otros animales, no reparando en que sea víbora, culebra, sapo o lagarto, y a falta de esto usan comer raíces, y algunas frutas salvajes' (1591, fol. 200v).

44 'tanto cuanto en su tierra son de valientes fuertes recios y muy sanos, por más malos mantenimientos que coman, y peores noches que lleven, y más desnudos y descalzos que anden, tanto son de miserables engeridos y enfermizos en viniendo a nuestro poder, y usando de regalo, y criándose como gente: quien viere un chichimeco hecho entre peñascos un demonio, y después le viere entre nosotros, hecho un mojigatillo, y vuelto un retrato de enfermedad y duelo, y que apenas le ha dado el dolorcito, o las camarillas, cuando al momento se muere' (1591, fol. 201v).

45 'por cuanto le quitan y privan de aquel natural sustento ... aunque de suyo es malísimo, para ellos es sano y muy bueno' (1591, fol. 202v).

46 'en su tierra estaban enseñados a correr y saltar por breñas y peñascos donde despedían y consumían con aquel exercicio fuerte todo mal humor' (1591, fol. 202v). For a discussion of Cortés's views on Chichimecs, see Gradie, 1994, 69.

brought to their city a result of their naturally very weak constitution ('son de naturaleza tan débil'),[47] Cárdenas would echo that view but rearranging its coordinates so as to make it not about a contrast between a European setting and the Americas but about the city, understood as a European space of civilisation, and the 'wilderness' beyond.

In earlier sections of the *Problemas y secretos* Cárdenas's description of Indigenous eating practices had been largely positive; Iberians were instead the consumers of (cooked) meat products and a variety of rich foods that negatively affected their health, while the diet of Indigenous people consisted mostly of wholesome 'chili peppers and corn tortillas' (1591, fol. 126r). But once the Chichimecs make an entrance in Book 3, their characterisation colours assessments of Indigenous bodies more generally. As Rebecca Earle has observed, differences in activity and diet were used by many writers of the period to emphasise the distance between Indigenous and European bodies in relation to humoral medical knowledge.[48] But unlike other sources written primarily for audiences in Spain, Cárdenas is careful to make food a consideration contingent upon a wider set of environmental factors, aware that by 1591 many foodstuffs and products formerly regarded as unfit for European consumption were making their way to their dining tables. He addressed this conundrum by discussing the ways in which substances like chocolate could be modified to suit European bodies. Book 2 of the *Problemas y secretos* centred precisely on this issue and articulated a staunch defence of the benefits of chocolate if mixed with other spices and matched to the drinker's constitution. Against writers like Acosta who denounced the deleterious effects of chocolate in broad strokes, 'for Cárdenas', Marcy Norton explains, 'the solution … was to promote proper use according to European medical principles in the classical tradition … he matched different types of chocolate preparations to individuals' humoral needs', an analytical framework that 'encapsulated the issues that propelled his whole book—defending and controlling the acculturation of Europeans in the Indies' (2008, 135). In that process, some Indigenous nourishment is made palatable, even exquisite, without closing the door altogether on using food to support abject readings of Indigenous mores.

Chichimecs are made into consumers of raw meat to dramatise their cultural savagery, with Cárdenas's phrasing veering off into examples of reptile and amphibian sources.[49] Indeed, the extent to which Chichimec

47 Quoted by Cook (1993, 224).

48 See in particular Earle's chapter, 'Humoralism and the colonial body' (2012, 19–53).

49 The rhetorical gesture of linking animals not common in Western diets to arguments of purported cultural superiority, and of exaggerating the scale of their consumption, has present-day iterations, as recently shown by some responses to the 2020 COVID-19 global pandemic. 'China is to blame', expressed, for example, US senator John Cornyn speaking to news outlets, 'because the culture where people eat bats and snakes and dogs and things like that, these viruses are transmitted from the animal to the people' (Slisco, 2020). See Earle for a discussion of sixteenth-century notions

bodies are marked as different forces Cárdenas to acknowledge the possible scepticism of his readers. They are presented as diametric opposites of Spaniards as much by what they consume as by what they do not, as, for example, water. 'They are able to sustain themselves throughout their entire lives without drinking water', Cárdenas will claim, recognising that the assertion might be hard for his readers to accept.[50] But he insists that is it a fact nonetheless, leading him to set aside the Chichimec body as a site of radical difference in comparison not just to Spaniards but to all of mankind: 'what for him is life is death for the rest of men'.[51]

'Ethnologically', as Charlotte Gradie notes, 'there was no one Chichimec people'; it was a label 'used by both Spanish and Nahuatl speakers to refer collectively to many different people who exhibited a wide range of cultural development from hunter-gatherers to sedentary agriculturists with sophisticated political organizations' (1994, 68). In colonial historiography, explains Amber Brian, 'they are depicted either as the progenitors of civilization in Anáhuac or as the nomadic barbarians of the northern frontier' (2017, 145). Chichimecs are mentioned in sources going back at least as far as Cortés's *Cartas de relación*, where he had singled them out as being 'very barbarous' and 'not so intelligent' compared to other indigenous groups (cited in Gradie, 1994, 69). Cárdenas's interest in writing about them would have been related to the end of the Chichimec War, an incursion lasting from 1555 to 1590, whereby the Spanish had attempted to control the northern indigenous groups of New Galicia and New Vizcaya (areas that today correspond to the states of Querétaro, San Luis Potosí, Aguascalientes, Guanajuato, Zacatecas and Jalisco). After decades-long unsuccessful attempts to subdue these groups by force, in the 1580s a different 'peace-by-purchase' strategy was adopted, providing food and clothing in exchange for assurances from them not to attack frontier settlers. Viceroy Luis de Velasco, *hijo*, to whom the *Problemas y secretos* is dedicated, would achieve the signing of a peace treaty the same year that Cárdenas's book was published, finally bringing the conflict to an end. Throughout the duration of the war, efforts to demonise Chichimecs had rehearsed the arguments that Cárdenas repeats, but his choice to continue advancing these ideas served a different function. For while the strongest contrasts between Spanish bodies and indigenous bodies do appear in the section focused on Chichimecs, it leads to a discussion about the nature of 'indios' more broadly that builds on the same ideas and imagery, extending the claims to groups who had little in common culturally or experientially with groups labelled as Chichimecs, and for whom *altepetl*, urban life would have been the norm.

on 'bestial foods', a label she draws from the writings of Francisco de Xerez, one of Francisco Pizarro's companions (2012, 66–67).

50 'La segunda propiedad que de ellos notamos es sustentarse toda la vida sin beber' (1591, fol. 203v).

51 'lo que para él es vida sea muerte para los demás hombres' (1591, fol. 203v).

Cárdenas's efforts to insulate and separate the Spanish body from the Indigenous body then turns to medicine for support, pathologising ethnic difference through an association with *bubas*.[52] In Hispanic sources, the first references that linked the disease to the Americas had appeared in Columbian documents from the Second Voyage and in Fray Ramón Pané's *Antigüedades de los indios* [Antiquities of the Indians], a source composed in the last years of the fifteenth century that explained *bubas* in the context of Taíno mythology. However, there was not a consensus in sixteenth-century Spain on its origins. Highly influential sources, such as Juan Fragoso's *Cirugía universal*, first published in Seville in 1581, had sided with the view that *morbo gálico* was not a new disease and subscribed instead to the idea that the illness could arise in different places simultaneously and was likely to also transfer by means other than physical contact. But Cárdenas rejects the possibility of a European origin and identifies it as an unquestionably American disease, linked to the original inhabitants of the region and prone to spread to other populations with similar humoral constitutions:

> There are contagious sicknesses that agree more with some types and complexions than with others, for the similarities that they have with them, and in the same manner the *bubas* have this property or affinity of being found in dirty and filth-ridden subjects; which is why we ordinarily find and see this illness start in Blacks, Indians, *mulatos*, and people who have a mix of the land, because all of these for the most part live with little cleanliness and restraint. … they cast from themselves an insufferable stench, mostly the Black and the Indian, who of their own nature are dirty bodies.[53]

52 'Syphilis', a term coined in an epic poem in 1530 by physician Girloamo Fracastoro, in not used by the medical writers of sixteenth-century Mexico who refer to *bubas* and, in the case of Farfán, both to *bubas* and *mal francés* [French disease]. Syphilis would be increasingly used with an equivalent meaning, however, even though today it is believed more than one kind of infection could have been described by these terms in early modern texts. The choice of terminology to name the disease is not unimportant, as it provides readers with a window into European attitudes where illness was also used to demarcate *naciones*. Germans called it *franzosenkrankheit* [French malady], the French called it *mal de Naples* [Neapolitan disease], the Dutch, Spanish scabies, and in Africa, India and Japan, it was called *mankabassam*, or Portuguese sickness.

53 'hay males contagiosos que frisan y simbolizan más con unos sujetos y complexiones que con otras, por la semejanza que con ellos tienen, de la misma suerte las bubas tienen esta propiedad o amistad de conservarse y hallarse siempre en sujetos sucios y llenos de inmundicia; por el cual respecto vemos de ordinario hallarse y comenzar este mal por negros, indios, mulatos y gente que tiene mezcla de la tierra, porque todos estos por la mayor parte viven con poca limpieza y recato. … echan de sí un insufrible hedor, mayormente el negro y el indio, que de su propia naturaleza son cuerpos sucios' (1591, fol. 196r, fol. 197r).

Although elsewhere Cárdenas establishes contrasts between Spanish and Indigenous bodies giving the latter an advantage, such as the rarity with which he claims they suffer from colds or urinary problems (1591, fol. 217r), the inferior condition of non-European bodies is made manifest in their propensity to transmittable diseases, not just with regards to *bubas* but also in the case of 'cocoliste [which] is a kind of pestilence that, being from this land, afflicts Indians and not Spaniards'.[54] As Jonathan Gil Harris notes, some sources blamed the spread of leprosy in Europe on 'the sexual contact between a Jew and a leper', and 'unlike other illnesses which were explained in exclusively humoral terms', writes Harris, 'leprosy had been frequently attributed throughout the Middle Ages to the pathogenic incursions of foreign bodies—particularly Jews' (2006, 27). The modern distinction between infection and contagion, Lawrence I. Conrad and Dominik Wujastyk remind us, does not map neatly onto ideas about disease transmission in the ancient and early modern worlds. Both Latin and Arabic understandings of *contagio* and *ʿadwā* 'encompass[ed] notions of touch, transmission, and transitiveness' referring to an illness, but they also conveyed a sense of 'transmissibility in general, [including] transmission through heredity (Conrad and Wujastyk, 2017, x). Under this light, the *Problemas y secretos* can be seen as a source that adapted and expanded on existing European understandings of communicative diseases, strengthening the hereditary aspect by linking it to negative assessments on a racialised 'other' in a New World context.

Like Fragoso, Benavides (see chapter 1) had argued two decades earlier that *bubas* had multiple causes and modes of transmission, which were not always venereal, something proven, according to him, by the fact that religious men of the highest repute sometimes became afflicted. Like Cárdenas, he linked the disease to non-European populations (to Africans in his case), but instead stressed factors such as the deleterious effects of a poor diet on human constitutions and volunteered no explicit judgments on the perceived moral shortcomings of these populations, even though the mention that dogs could also purportedly suffer terribly from the same illness did open the door for readers to make problematic inferences, such as bestiality. Benavides's tone had not resolved that ambiguity. Writing in the *Secretos* on how the illness affected Europeans living in Santo Domingo, he explained:

> The cause of this [*bubas*] is that those who are born in that land are given to Black women to nurse, since to date I have not seen any Spanish woman who nurses her children. They secure before giving birth a Black woman with the best milk … and after childbirth they give the child to the Black woman … and the children eat of the foodstuffs that the Black women and their own children eat (which are very bad nourishment) and as are the foods, so are the humours they engender. And these same Black

54 'el cocoliztle es un modo de pestilencia, que por ser propio de esta tierra, da a los indios, y no a los españoles' (1591, fol. 194v).

women and their children are all covered in *bubas*, from which it follows that those who interact and communicate with them have them too. And thus all who are born in that land do not have their perfect colour but are instead a *mulato* colour.[55]

Agustín Farfán (discussed in chapter 3), for his part, railed against the 'idiots' and the '*matasanos*' [slayers of the healthy] who tortured patients afflicted with *bubas* by subjecting them to ineffective cures that only increased their suffering. For him, the illness had many causes and was not necessarily of American origin, even if one possible cause echoed Benavides's explanation associating *bubas* with non-Spanish bodies: 'you may give this syrup (as I have said) to pregnant women', writes Farfán, 'and to the children, mostly in this land, because they suffer from this disease, because their mothers hand them over to Indigenous women, and to *mulatas*, and nowadays to Chichimeca women, to avoid doing the work (of nursing) themselves.'[56] Although not entirely clear from his phrasing, Farfán's position is arguably more invested in suggesting contagion by way of physical proximity with afflicted people, or with groups socially scapegoated as carriers of the disease at the time, than in putting forth unequivocal judgments on their purported bodily inferiority. For Farfán, contact with Indigenous and African-descended wet-nurses was one of several possible ways of contracting the disease, but it was not singled out in any special way, afforded the same textual space as other possibilities. Importantly, he prescribes the syrup not just to the children but to their Spanish mothers, criticising the women's nursing practices but decoupling the transmission of the illness from the consumption of breast milk. His ambiguous stance on this point is further complicated by another passage on the health benefits of breast milk for adult patients in the context of Indigenous women.[57]

55 'la causa dello es que los que nacen en aquella tierra danlos a criar a las negras, porque hasta ahora no he visto que ninguna española críe a sus hijos. Previénense antes que paran de una negra que tenga la mejor leche … y luego que paren entregan la criatura a la negra … y las criaturas comen de los manjares que coman las negras y sus hijos (que son muy malas comidas) y así cuales son las comidas, se engendran los humores. Y también las mismas negras, y sus hijos, todos están llenos de bubas, de lo cual es razón evidente que las han de tener los que tratan y comunican con ellas. Y así todos los que nacen en aquella tierra no tienen su perfecta color sino [que son] amulatados' (1567, fol. 9v).

56 'Puédese (como dije) dar este jarabe a mujeres preñadas, y a los niños, mayormente en esta tierra, porque padecen de este mal, porque sus madres los dan a criar a indias, y mulatas, y ahora en estos tiempos a las chichimecas, por no trabajar ellas' (1579, 220r).

57 Farfán writes: '[For hectic fevers] it is very good to have two wet-nurses, or *chichiguas*, which in Nahuatl means the same, and drink their milk to regain the youth of younger years … believe me it is an admirable cure' [con calentura hética es poderoso para tener dos amas, o chichiguas, que en lengua mexicana es lo mismo, y mamare la

The racially marked mentions of breast milk are eliminated in the 1595 edition of the *Tractado*; allusions to human milk as an ingredient with medicinal properties remain but no longer linked to any particular group. Instead, Farfán adds a section that is the closest he would come to affording Indigenous bodies a separate category, in a chapter with the heading 'To remove fevers in Indians' [Para quitar las calenturas a los Indios]. In this new section, Farfán described their preferred method for purging themselves, which he had characterised as sound in the first edition, now explaining it involved green verbena, not ruling it out for Spaniards (1579, 231r–231v; 1592, 179v). But rather than a discussion on bodily difference, the section instead offers a reflection on the difficulty of treating Indigenous patients due to cultural differences in eating habits. The text warns European practitioners against cures that involved bloodletting given Indigenous people's spartan diet: 'truly they do not tolerate many bloodlettings, for if in health they eat little, when sick they eat almost nothing … and die stricken with hunger and thirst'.[58]

Hinojosos went further than the others in linking the disease to a venereal mode of transmission but, like Farfán, he did not single out any *nación* as being especially prone to becoming infected. The fact that both Farfán and Hinojosos recommend Indigenous forms of treatment to their readers belies the idea that either one was persuaded by a model of consubstantial bodily difference between them. Moreover, in the case of Hinojosos, he would go as far as to argue for the opposite. In a section on paediatric medicine in the second edition, discussing the causes and treatments for *ahíto* (an inflammation of the large intestine), he explains that although Indigenous peoples and Africans are better at hiding their symptoms, their bodies are afflicted just like any other:

> [The signs of *ahito*] are clear: but note its true cause [which he has just described in the previous paragraph as stemming from feeding the baby too often] that even the Blacks and the Indians and any people at all, excuse themselves and deny that it afflicts them, but it cannot be hidden regardless of how young the patient is, as the belching is so great, and the fever so excessive that it is nearly as bad as typhus, and these sufferings can lead to smallpox.[59]

leche dellas volviendo a la primera edad … y créanme que es remedio admirable] (1579, 264r).

58 'Y verdaderamente los indios no sufren muchas sangrías, porque en salud comen poco, y enfermos casi nada … Y cierto que los más de ellos se mueren traspasados de hambre y de sed' (1595, fol. 179v).

59 'Son bien manifiestas [las señales del ahíto]: mas note que es la causa, que hasta los negros e indios, y cualquier gente que sea, se excusan y niegan el ahitarse, mas no lo pueden tener secreto por chiquito que sea el que se ahitó, porque son tan grandes regueldos y tan excesiva la calentura, que no hay tabardete que le haga ventaja, y destos ardores suelen dar viruelas' (1595, fol. 179v).

Rather than insist on differences, Hinojosos finds correspondences between the bodies of Indigenous subjects and those of Spaniards, which comes into focus in the 1595's *Svmma*'s account of a public autopsy carried out at the request of authorities to investigate the effects of smoking on the internal organs:

> In the year 1592, the 7th of January, a citizen of Oaxaca died, and before most of his fellow citizens, and at the insistence of the surgeons, the mayor, who was Luis Xuárez de Peralta at the time, ordered that he be opened, because it had been said that he was an avid smoker of *picietl*, and in the interest of the public good, he ordered his body opened, and I was present, and I saw that his body was like those on which I had performed dissections seventeen years before, when the great cocoliste had occurred, because his liver was very swollen, and his lungs dry and black, and his spleen very large and hard, and his intestines black and in pieces.[60]

There is an important slippage in the comparison between the ravages of smoking and those of cocoliste. Indeed, as we already saw, earlier in his career Hinojosos had treated many cases of cocoliste and had had ample opportunity to see how it devastated the internal organs of the patients that succumbed to it. Yet the bodies that set the coordinates and the basis for a comparison were by and large not those of Europeans or *criollos*, but of Indigenous men and women. In his original retelling of the incident, Hinojosos had praised the bravery of the priests and lay religious men who in 1576 had gone out into the Indigenous communities afflicted by the epidemic to bring aid and offer assistance: 'And thus went those who desired the health of mankind among the sick, not shying away from the occasion despite it being serious and contagious, but delving deeper in it, wanting more the salvation of the Indians' souls than their own health.'[61] Although Hinojosos did note that the communities affected were 'the Blacks and Chichimec Indians [to such an extent that] Mexico, and the mines, and all of New Spain was left almost without service',[62] these men's valour lay precisely in choosing to expose

60 'El año de mil y quinientos y noventa y dos, a siete de enero, murió un ciudadano de Oaxaca, y a contemplación de los de más ciudadanos, y a pedimiento de los cirujanos; lo mandó abrir el alcalde mayor, que al presente era Luis Suárez de Peralta, porque le dijeron que era gran chupador de humo de piciete, y con el deseo y bien común lo mandó abrir, y yo me hallé presente, y vi que estaba su cuerpo como los que yo había hecho anatomía; diez y seis años antes; cuando el gran cocoliste, porque tenía el hígado muy hinchado, y los livianos secos y prietos, y el bazo muy grande y duro, y las tripas prietas y a trechos' (1595, fols. 150v–151r).

61 'Y así andaban los deseosos de la salud del género humano entre los enfermos, no huyendo de la ocasión aunque era grave y contagiosa, sino metiéndose en ella, queriendo más la salvación de las almas de los naturales que su misma salud' (1977, 208).

62 'en ese propio tiempo se murieron muchos negros e indios chichimecos, que quedó México y las minas y toda la Nueva España casi sin servicio' (1977, 210).

themselves to the risk of contagion. Cárdenas's claims of Spanish immunity to cocoliste are nowhere to be found in the source closest to a recollection of that event. Tellingly, Farfán does not address cocoliste separately, opting to discuss contagious illnesses that exhibited similar symptoms in sections on 'tabardete' [typhus] and 'calentura pestilencial' [epidemic fever], neither of which are racially marked in the *Tractado*.

Hinojosos's failure to engage with a model such as the one proposed by Cárdenas is perhaps unsurprising if we consider his chief place of employment was, after all, the Hospital Real de los Naturales. Despite the fact that in the *Svmma*, barring the episode on cocoliste, dissected bodies are not marked ethnically and are easily assumed to be of European descent by readers, the majority of the bodies the author would have had access to over the course of a lifelong career would have been those of his patients, in a hospital that tended chiefly to Indigenous people. In the *Svmma*'s first-hand description of structures and processes, whose bodies are we really seeing? Stripped of skin and of cultural or ethnic markers, could the image in the 1595 edition not also be read as the depiction of an Indigenous subject? Even if we move past the counterfeit dimension of the image to regard it as an amalgamated representation of a canonical body, designed primarily as a mirror to be used by Spaniards, we are still left with the question of what makes the Indigenous body a good enough stand-in on which to study information about human physiology. What are the limits to that correspondence?

There is one more intriguing detail in Hinojosos's text supporting the notion of a New World medical body template that belies a multi-ethnic experiential basis, found in his discussion on tumours and tears in men's testicles. After describing different scenarios that might cause these problems, there is a brief aside instructing practitioners on the correct course of action 'if authorities ever ordered removing the testicles, that it should be done in this manner' (fol. 64v). The process entailed tying the sack loosely, cutting the skin with a knife, severing the sack with scissors, tying the skin with waxed string, cauterising the area with a hot iron, sewing the wound and then follow-up care using a method already described for healing fresh wounds. Hinojosos ends the section as he often does, by alluding to his own practice: 'this is the safest way of removing testicles, and I have removed some, and it has gone very well' (fol. 64v). Although there is limited evidence to suggest that Spanish or Indigenous bodies were subjected to castration as a form of punishment in New Spain,[63] there are indications that it may have been a condoned, if not commonplace, practice applied to Africans. As Nicolás Ngou-Mve has found, in a letter to the Council of the Indies dated October 1579, the same viceroy Martín Enríquez, mentioned earlier

63 See, for example, Zeb Tortorici's analysis of a Mayan boy tried for bestiality in Mérida in 1563 and sentenced to banishment and castration (2018, 125–27). Tortorici's archival research does not find evidence of other tried cases where castration was used as punishment, and suggests it could have been an isolated occurrence.

in relation to Hernández and the cocoliste response, recalled what seemed to him better days when delinquent *negros* and *mulatos* in New Spain could still be threatened with castration, and lamented that the practice had since been supressed by the king (1999, 13). A direct consultation of the document in question supports Ngou-Mve's conclusion that it may not have been an uncommon practice, considering Enríquez's choice of phrasing which suggests a routine occurrence given his preference for the imperfect verb tense: 'the punishment that was usually administered during the eras of don Luis de Mendoza and don Luis de Velasco was to castrate them, which they feared terribly, and it was done until some years after my arrival' (1579, fols. 1v–2r).[64] Enríquez had for some time expressed misgivings about Black populations in New Spain and, despite community-organised attempts to persuade authorities to build a hospital to care for them separately, the concern that these facilities would become spaces of resistance had thwarted their efforts. In a prior letter, dated 28 April 1572, also brought to light by Ngou-Mve's work, Enríquez is unequivocal on the reasons behind his reservations:

> The *mulatos* have also brought a document (*cédula*) from Your Highness in which they demand, barring any objections, that a hospital be constructed where they may cure themselves by means of their own assemblies and brotherhoods. … I have never accepted the construction of another hospital for Blacks (*destinado a negros*): we should all go together, because all of us: Spaniards, *mestizos*, *negros* and *mulatos*, speak the same tongue. … It is necessary for Blacks who become ill to be cured by their masters, for if not done in this way, it would create an opportunity for two thousand Blacks to come together, perhaps more.[65]

Seen in its historical context, Hinojosos's textual descriptions of a New World body stand at the edge of what in the late sixteenth century becomes a colonial paradox, with European discourses on physiology gathering the strength to form a scientific basis for the articulation of irreconcilable differences among bodies belonging to different *naciones*, and anatomy initially resisting that pull as it gravitated towards surgery's new questions on what form could reveal about function above other considerations. Neither Farfán nor Hinojosos feel compelled to racialise the New World body, and it is telling that there are few to no *mestizos* or *mulatos* singled out as subjects of particular interest in their discussions on human anatomy or physiology. In contrast, Cárdenas's choice to also deny them room in the *Problemas* operates differently given the resonance of the moments where he does acknowledge them: the quick mention of *mulatos* already cited and the two

64 'la pena que se les solía dar [en] el tiempo de don Luis de Mendoza y don Luis de Velasco que era caparlos, lo cual temían terriblemente, y se efectuaba hasta algunos años después que yo vine allegado'.

65 Cited by Ngou-Mve (1999, 14) in Spanish.

instances when he employs circumlocution to avoid conjuring *mestizos* unto the page, referring to them instead as 'people with a mix of the land' [*gente con mezcla de la tierra*].[66]

Medicine and its ideas about human bodies at the end of a century where Europeans had struggled to find their moorings through unprecedented territorial expansion and colonisation proved an unsteady platform from which to engage issues of social stratification. These challenges would ultimately come not from science or medicine but from moral and political philosophy. And yet allusions to a physical body understood in physiological and anatomical terms became a constant point of reference for the major voices in the philosophical and literary arenas of the seventeenth century, from Miguel del Cervantes to Lope de Vega to René Descartes. At the start of this new era, on a European stage and before audiences ushering in a century that would be defined as much by scientific progress as by never-before-seen levels of racialised exploitation at the expense of brown and Black bodies, a fictional Jewish character pleaded for equal treatment on the basis of a medicalised bodily experience. Did people belonging to different *naciones* not have the same 'hands, organs, dimensions, senses, affections, [were] fed with the same food, hurt with the same weapons, [were] subject to the same diseases [or were] healed by the same means'?[67] Meanwhile, the authors of the two most read locally printed medical books in New Spain—Hinojosos, the nurse practitioner, and Farfán, a *radicado* doctor whose work we now turn to—were each coming to the end of long medical careers, built across a very different demographic environment, where they had unremarkably cared for their patients as if it were so.

66 In addition to the passage cited, Cárdenas also uses the phrase when describing the physical appearance and personality of the Spaniard of the Indies. Commenting on their skin colour, Cárdenas offers that the Spaniards of the Indies, young as well as old, are 'generally white and ruddy (so long as they do not have a mix of the land), and are also frank, liberal, happy, energetic, affable' ['porque todos en general son blancos y colorados (como no tengan mezcla de la tierra) son asimismo francos, liberales, recocijados, animosos, afables'], fol. 179r.

67 Shylock's dialogue in Act III, scene I of Shakespeare's *The Merchant of Venice*, composed between 1596 and 1597 (Shakespeare, 2005, 466).

CHAPTER 3

Weakening the sex

The medicalisation of female gender identity in New Spain

In the surgical and anatomical books written in Europe during the sixteenth century the bodies studied and described were, by and large, those of men.[1] Medical authors could recommend adapting a given procedure to the needs of a female patient so as to account for a difference in body mass, or treatments could be modified to suit a woman's colder and wetter temperament, but the description of bodily structures and substances not directly linked to generation—bile, bones, eyes—these were generally not marked as female. Male templates were preferred when it came to illustrating information that would apply to both sexes for 'anatomy', as Katharine Park observes, 'was about knowing the generic human body, which was understood as male' (2006, 14).[2] Therapeutic care relating to women's fertility and successful procreation had been an important topic in medieval medicine, and texts such as the *De passionibus mulierum* [On the diseases of women] circulated widely in Europe from the twelfth to the fifteenth centuries. But in the context of early modern Iberia, relatively few books focusing solely on women's medicine would be printed, with discussions on female physiology and anatomy usually circumscribed to their reproductive function in larger, more established

1 This chapter builds on archival research findings on Hinojosos I first shared at Queen's University Belfast in November 2013, in the paper 'The local doctor? Medical writing in Mexico from 1578–1610'. The discussion on Juan Fragoso draws on research findings presented at the University of St Andrews in July 2017, in the paper 'Sound, scale and human-animal distress in early modern Hispanic medical writing'.

2 Although present-day research in genetics and biology has called into question the division of humans into only two sexes, with some biologists arguing for five (Fausto-Sterling) and other scholars proposing instead a spectrum model (Ainsworth), early modern social and biological categories in Europe and colonial America used male and female as its two main classificatory groups. Cases of individuals who did not fully conform to period expectations of what constituted a male or a female due to physical traits, gender expression, sexual attraction or other considerations tended to be described in relation to this binary division and not as asexual or *sui generis* bodies, as will be discussed later in the chapter.

texts about general medicine or surgery.[3] Their textual underrepresentation initially extended to New Spain as well. Neither Bravo's *Opera medicinalia* (1570), Hinojosos's first edition of the *Svmma* (1578) nor Agustín Farfán's own first edition of his *Tractado breve de anothomia y chirvgia, y de algvnas enfermedades, que mas comunmente suelen hauer en esta Nueua España* [Brief treatise on anatomy and surgery, and on some common illnesses found in this New Spain] (1579), as the first three texts printed in the New World that dealt with anatomy and physiology, showed a particular interest in ailments afflicting women. Mentions were made, but these were integrated alongside other subjects. However, by the 1590s the situation had changed. Albeit in passing, Cárdenas in the *Problemas y secretos* (1591) offered a comparative assessment of the physiological processes experienced by women in the Indies versus their counterparts in Europe, and the second editions of both Farfán's *Tractado*, from 1592, and Hinojosos's *Svmma*, from 1595, were revised so as to make way for information on women's health, material that was organised into distinct stand-alone sections in the case of the latter.[4] Hinojosos's and Farfán's joint departure from the norm affords a particularly useful opportunity for scholars of early colonial Latin America. First, as authors who were writing at the same place and time, and who both published first and second, revised editions separated by roughly the same number of years, juxtaposing their respective outputs creates a focused snapshot of how medicine viewed women's bodies during the viceroyalty's period of consolidation while elucidating the extent to which medical sources reflected (and quite possibly informed) colonial discourse on gender more broadly. Secondly, and perhaps even more importantly, a close reading of these materials opens a new window into the lives of early colonial women, for nowhere in New World print culture at this point in time had women received such sustained, ample discussion as

3 *De passionibus mulierum* [On the diseases of women] was a text attributed to Trota of Salerno, a female physician from twelfth-century southern Italy, though the materials that would come to circulate as the 'Trotula' are thought to be the work of at least three distinct writers (Green, 2002, xii). At least two manuals on midwifery are known to have been published in Spain in the sixteenth century, one by Damián Carbón and another by Francisco Núnez, as will be discussed later in this chapter.

4 As with Hinojosos's text, there will be small changes to the title of the second and third editions of Farfán's book, which appeared in 1592 as the *Tractado brebe de medicina, y de todas las enfermedades* [Brief treatise on medicine, and on all illnesses], and again in 1610 as *De medicina y de todas las enfermedades* [On medicine and on all illnesses]. Slight variations in how scholars refer to the first edition are partly due to the fact that the title page has been lost in one of the three surviving copies of the book (the one at the Biblioteca Nacional de México) and later sections are not consistent in how they name the text. The copies at the Bancroft Library and the Huntington Library do retain their title pages which helps to settle the matter. Each printing featured a different image on its title page: an image of Saint Augustine holding a church in 1579, an image of a friar thought by some to be a portrait of the author in 1592, and a smaller image of Saint Augustine in 1610.

in these medical sources. A tangential consideration at best in early Mexican and Peruvian imprints, medical literature unexpectedly brings women into the limelight.[5]

The shift in focus is likely to have been less a question of science than of an evolving social reality and demographics. European women had first arrived in the Americas in 1498 as part of Columbus's third voyage and, although initially rates of immigration were low, with only around 1,000 women coming from Spain between 1509 and 1538, according to Susan Migden Socolow, by mid-century they comprised a significant portion of the colonising population (2014, 57–58). The rate of immigration of Spanish women during the second half of the sixteenth century would reach 'a high point of 28 to 40 percent of all immigrants ... declining slightly by the seventeenth century' (Socolow, 2014, 62); this change in the male to female ratio is reflected in local medical texts. Women were part of a larger venture for laying the foundations of viceregal societies, and the Spanish Crown encouraged their emigration considering them more stable purveyors of culture. As Socolow explains, they 'were seen as "civilizers"; it was they who would teach proper behavior and social forms to their menfolk ... Indeed, [they] were a metaphor for rootedness' (2014, 57). Thus, discussions on women's health likely had urgent implications, as not only were they a necessary tool for the biological viability of Hispanic societies in the Americas, the very success and stability of the colonial enterprise itself was linked to their roles as pillars of European value systems. But were these women (and their bodies) up to the task?

Despite Cárdenas's detailed explanation on the positive transformative power of New World environments on Spaniards as a *nación* (discussed in chapter 2), his remarks dealing specifically with women are more ambiguous. In the *Problemas y secretos*, he had asked readers to compare just how different Spaniards from Spain were from those of the Indies, selecting a man born in Spain and one born locally as contrasting examples, finding in favour of the

5 Bartolomé de las Casas can be said to counter this trend, as he mentions Indigenous women frequently in his texts. Las Casas tended to portray them as young victims of abuse or as defenceless mothers of young children, in an effort to draw sympathy for the plight of native communities. Women of European descent, however, did not receive any special mention. Bernal Díaz del Castillo discusses the figure of Malinche in the *Historia verdadera de la conquista de la Nueva España* [True account of the conquest of New Spain] (Madrid, 1632), composed in Guatemala around 1568, but again women are not a salient topic in the work as a whole. In the context of early Mexican imprints, Fray Alonso de la Vera Cruz's *Speculum conjugiorum*, printed by Juan Pablos in 1556, necessarily addressed the topic of women given that work's focus on the institution of marriage in relation to canon law and conversion. Assessments about women and the policing of their behaviour likely circulated more abundantly in New Spain's manuscript culture, particularly after the foundation of the first convent in 1540.

latter. At the end of that passage, Cárdenas adds one more line that would extend the same positive conclusion to women:

> let a woman from Spain come now and enter into a conversation with many ladies from the Indies, and immediately it becomes clear and known that she is from Spain due to the advantage that the people born in the Indies have over those of us who come from Spain in their demeanour and speech: for should they decide to pay a compliment, extend an invitation or outline a well-reasoned and timely argument that, forsooth, there is no courtier born in Madrid or Toledo that can compose it better, or make it more refined.[6]

Although plainly referring to women initially in the passage, by the end of the sentence, the phrasing becomes labyrinthine, and he seems to be referring once again to the 'Spaniards of the Indies' in general terms. Unlike in the previous section, there is no underlying scientific explanation enlisting humoral medicine here to justify the eloquence of female subjects similar to the one he had offered for men. This absence presents a problem if we recall that, for Cárdenas, the wet and cold nature of the New World tempered the dry and hot constitution of the choleric male Spaniard, bringing him into a beneficial choleric-sanguine state. However, women's cold and wet humoral makeup would give rise instead to a deleterious effect, and while Cárdenas decides not to rehearse that argument in this passage, he does address it in the section of the *Problemas y secretos* discussing women's physiology directly. There, Cárdenas finds that unlike their male counterparts, the bodies of European women in New Spain were weakened by their new surroundings and rendered more susceptible to vices, such as dirt eating.

While not a phenomenon exclusive to Spain, there are several representations of 'dirt eaters' in Golden Age literature, where, along with the practice of drinking steel-water, ingesting clay appears as a method for lightening the colour of the skin and could also suggest an effort to end an unwanted pregnancy.[7] Cárdenas makes no mention of dirt eating as an abortifacient,

6 'pues venga ahora una mujer de España, y entre en conversación de muchas damas de las Indias, al momento se diferencia y conoce ser de España, sólo por la ventaja que en cuanto al trascender, y hablar nos hace la española gente nacida en Indias, a los que de España venimos, pues póngase a decir un primor, un ofrecimiento, o una razón bien limada y sacada de punto, mejor viva yo que haya cortesano criado dentro de Madrid o Toledo, que mejor la lime y la componga' (1591, fols. 177r–177v).

7 More attention has been paid by critics to the link between dirt eating and women's chastity than to how the practice may reflect anxieties over miscegenation in Iberian contexts that privileged whiteness, whether in America or in Europe, and set against different sets of populations perceived as darker-skinned in either case. On the link between dirt eating and abortion, Albarracín Teulón (1954) cites a passage from *El esclavo fingido* [The disguised slave] (c. 1599–1603), a play attributed by some to Lope de Vega, where it reads: 'Avoid the woman who eats half a jar, as she does it

but does refer to the cosmetic context in his explanation as to why the 'Spanish women of this land' [*las españolas mujeres de esta tierra*] had recurring problems with their menses:

> The first reason is that all of the women and ladies of the Indies, mostly those of New Spain, are given to this vice of eating dirt, clay, cocoa and similar filth, that not only do not nourish the body, but as things composed of thick, earthy and sedimentary substances, they close and block their inner vessels in terrible fashion. One could wonder why the women of this land are more prone to eating dirt and cocoa than those of other provinces; I answer that many do so out of sheer viciousness, wanting only in this to achieve a lighter skin colour (which they call a ladies' colour).[8]

In contrast to the positive judgment offered earlier when discussing the humoral constitution of Spaniards in New Spain, his depiction of women as more prone to vice undermines that assessment. However, while his explanation suggests a failure in the proper policing of the behaviour of women who wilfully choose to ingest what he deems toxic substances, Cárdenas identifies an underlying physiological reason for their actions that recuperates Hippocratic tradition and realigns its parameters to the local social context:

> The second cause [of women's dirt eating] is the constitution of the Indies in this manner: given that in the Indies there is an overabundance of phlegmatic and cold humidity, and [women's] wombs are of the same complexion, all the excrements and thick, slow and cold humours accumulate in the veins and vessels of the aforementioned womb.[9]

not for the clay but because her womb is a vessel, and though the doctor comes to cure her of her sickly color, she is healed by the midwife') ['Reniega tú de mujer / que se come medio jarro / que no lo hace por el barro, / sino por dar a entender / que la barriga es (vasera), / y con enfermo color / entra a curalla el doctor / y sánala la partera'] (1954, 213). On this topic, see also Morel-Fatio (1972), Pérez Marín (2003) and López-Terrada (2014). For a discussion of the topic in the context of enslaved Africans in the Anglo Caribbean and the Antebellum South, see part II of Hogarth's *Medicalizing Blackness* (2017). For a discussion of the practice of drinking steel water in Golden Age Spain, see Ambrosi and De Beni (2014).

8 'la primera causa es, el ser todas las mujeres y señoras de las Indias, mayormente las de la Nueva España, dadas a este vicio de comer tierra, barro, cacao y semejantes inmundicias, las cuales no sólo no les dan sustento al cuerpo, pero como cosas compuestas de sustancia gruesa terrestre y feculenta, cierran y opilan terriblemente las sobredichas vías y vasos. Pero podría alguno preguntar, por qué causa, más las mujeres de esta tierra, que otras de diferentes provincias fuesen dadas a comer tierra y cacao, respondo que muchas lo hacen de puro vicio, pretendiendo totalmente con esto, traer quebrado el color (que llaman color de damas)' (1591, fols. 216r–216v).

9 'La segunda causa es el temple de las Indias en esta forma, como en las Indias abunda tanta suma de humedad flemática y fría, y la matriz de su naturaleza sea de la misma complexión, acuden todos los excrementos y humores gruesos lentos y fríos a las mismas venas y vasos de la dicha matriz' (1591, fol. 216v).

According to the *Problemas y secretos*, while in Europe the land enjoyed more temperate degrees of heat and dryness, New Spain, with its abundant cold and phlegmatic humidity, mirrored women's inner constitution, exacerbating their weakness of character and leaving them more vulnerable before illness. Women were accountable for their actions, and he does make it a point to state that the Spanish women of Peru fared better because they behaved themselves with more restraint than those in New Spain and were less prone to dirt eating and chocolate drinking. But in their case as well, that was true only up to a certain point, seeing as the bodies they inhabited could not help but fail them and lead them to make poor choices. In Cárdenas's scientifically reasoned model, the female Spaniards of the Americas, particularly those in Mexico, would be even less fit than their counterparts in the Peninsula to actively participate in the decision-making arena of the viceroyalties, or to assume leading roles in their political governance.[10]

Just how different were women's bodies to those of men in the medical sources of early colonial Latin America, and what information do the work of writers like Cárdenas reveal about period notions on matters of gender and sexuality? Hinojosos's description of fetal development in the second edition of the *Svmma* provides a clue. The first edition of the text, published originally in 1578, had a total of 201 octavo folios divided into seven sections: on anatomy, artificial bloodletting, abscesses, fresh wounds, *bubas*, fractures and dislocations, and pestilence; the first part was the lengthiest of all extending over 17 chapters. In contrast, the 1595 version expanded the work into 204 quarto folios (a 4to in 8s edition), almost doubling it in size, and organised the material into 11 parts instead: on rheum,[11] anatomy, artificial bloodletting, abscesses, *opilaciones*,[12] fresh wounds, fractures and dislocations, *tabardete* and cocoliste, childbirth, paediatric care and antidotes. In the second printing, the section on anatomy was condensed into 12 chapters, and three of its new sections dealt either primarily or substantially with women's health. In the fourth chapter of Book 9 from that version, Hinojosos offered a

10 Encarnación Juárez-Almendros makes a similar point in her work on discursive representations of women in early modern Spain, arguing for the female body to be understood as one rendered disabled. See in particular chapter 1 of *Disabled Bodies in Early Modern Spanish Literature* (2017, 17–55). Read in this light, Cárdenas's own model did more than appropriate Iberian views: it enlisted science to strengthen their reach in ways that further bolstered the legitimacy of the patriarchy in an overseas context.

11 For Hinojosos, rheum was a watery substance produced in the brain out of vapors that arose from the generative organs, and which served to lubricate joints. It could aid in dissolving obstructions which the patient then released in his or her urine (1595, fols. 4v–5r).

12 'Oppilations' (also documented to have been used as a term in period English) were obstructions in the flow of the body's humoral substances, and a condition which women were particularly prone to in the early modern imagination.

description of the process of conception. According to him, 'the seeds of the man and the woman are joined in the womb of the mother, where they are nourished for six days', after which point they are covered by 'a little fabric' so that 'they do not become separated, for from each little breadcrumb of the seeds a child, or a monster will be born, just like the number of cups one adds of milk in a recipe determines how much custard will be made'.[13] 'After nine days', the text continues, 'this little fabric becomes red, like cochineal, and three little cavities arise the size of garbanzo beans which are the three principal members, and they begin to communicate with one another', forming the brain, the heart and the rest of the organs.[14] Similes and diminutives allow Hinojosos to achieve a higher level of precision in his narrative, with bodily structures resembling foodstuffs, and the gestation of a child organised as a culinary recipe. However, as the passage advances, and despite providing the exact timing of developmental changes, the language is less clear on the matter of sex differentiation:

> If at thirty days there is enough heat and other dispositions are in place, God endows [the child] with a soul and [he] is a man; and if one degree of heat is missing, [the child] turns out female and manly who speaks like a man, and has manly traits, and if there is a lack of heat, it happens at sixty days; and if when it comes time for the quickening, heat rises by one degree, [the child] becomes a man, and is an effeminate man, who speaks like a woman.[15]

Although Hinojosos claims to have discerned this information from the direct observation of the cadaver of 'a woman killed three or four months into her pregnancy [in whom] all this I saw at which I marvelled',[16] the fact that it is possible to trace his ideas to Iberian period sources allows us to bring a number of elements into focus, and to discern that he has made a slight mistake, neglecting to mention the case of the non-manly woman.

13 'Las dos simientes del varón, y de la mujer se juntan en un seno de la madre, y se están fomentando por seis días, al cabo de los cuales se pone blanca como leche, y le cubre una telica ... para que no se apartasen las simientes, porque de cada migajita de estas simientes, se criaría un niño, o un monstruo, así como la leche después de echado el cuajo, cuantas escudillas de aquella leche saliese tanta serían de cuajada' (1595, fol. 168v).

14 'al cabo de nueve días, se pone esta túnica colorada como una grana: y luego se hacen tres vejiguitas, como tres garbanzos que son los tres miembros principales, y luego se comienzan a comunicar sus virtudes' (1595, fol. 168v).

15 'si a los treinta días tiene calor bastante y las demás disposiciones necesarias, infunde Dios el ánima, y es hombre; y si le falta un grado de calor sale mujer y hombruda que habla como hombre, y tiene condiciones de hombre, y si hay falta de calor, pasa a los sesenta días; y si al tiempo de animar, sube un grado de calor, se hace hombre, y es amarionado, que habla como mujer' (1595, fols. 168v–169r).

16 'En una mujer que mataron preñada de tres o cuatro meses, vi todo esto que me admiré' (1595, fol. 169r).

Hinojosos, as did most of the medical sources circulating in Spain at the time, conceived of sex as a continuum, where 'men' and 'women' were presented as normative sex identities occupying distinct positions along a spectrum that also admitted transitional categories. 'To be a woman or a man', as Richard Cleminson and Francisco Vázquez García explain, 'was not so much to possess a particular biological quality but rather to display a social attribute', creating a context where 'the distinction between sex and gender was meaningless [within] the "heterosexual matrix" of the period' (2013, 6–7).[17] In ways that do not map onto later or current understandings of sexual and gender identities, men (a concept akin to what today could be deemed cisgender heterosexual males) and women (likewise understood as a marker similar to cisgender heterosexual females) were seen as analogous but distinct ontological categories against which other positions were measured, including bearded women, lactating men, manly women, men who sought out other men,[18] men who turned into women or women who turned into men.

17 One of the best-known recent attempts to study early modern sex and gender is Thomas Laqueur's one-sex model, which argues that prior to the mid eighteenth century, there were 'many genders, but only one adaptable sex' (1990, 35). This model has been strongly criticised by other scholars, most notably by Katharine Park and Robert Nye, who accuse Laqueur of imposing a 'false homogeneity on his sources' and of using anachronistic understandings of sex and gender to view the premodern era (Park & Nye, 1991, 54–55). Cleminson and Vázquez García take into account these critiques, Park's in particular, but still deem Laqueur's "one-sex model" useful to discuss the early modern Iberian context. While my own work benefits greatly from clarifications emerging from this conversation, it deliberately avoids entering into it given the challenge posed by current interdisciplinary research in biology and the social sciences questioning the scientific basis of sexual dimorphism, an assumption underpinning most existing scholarship on early modern sexuality. As the work of Anne Fausto-Sterling and Claire Ainsworth has shown, despite prevailing social attitudes and dominant legal systems that define sex in binary terms, emerging research over the last 30 years on DSD (Differences of Sex Development) populations, such as individuals with Klinefelter Syndrome, Congenital Adrenal Hyperplasia or Androgen Insensitivity Syndrome and, more recently, on the role of genes like SRY, WNT4 and RSPO1 (rather than chromosomal karyotypes alone) in the fetal development of gonads, challenge the scientific basis of such classification. Although dismissed in the past as medical anomalies that did not necessarily compromise a male/female model, or grouped under the category of 'intersex', current studies on biology and human genetics underscore both the recurrence as well as the considerable percentage of human populations reflecting such traits in their genetic makeup over time on a global scale. My analysis therefore strives to adhere as closely as possible to the categories and the language present in the sixteenth-century sources being examined without attempting to map them onto either biological or social understandings of sex and gender today. See in particular Ainsworth (2015, 288–91) and Fausto-Sterling (2012, 3–11).

18 Same-sex attraction is indicated in different ways, as evidenced in the passages cited in this chapter, and usually by invoking a euphemism rather than by describing a sex

This model allowed for a degree of flexibility in determining the sex of an individual but insisted at the same time on the attribution of a predominant sexual identity that would correspond to a rigid heterosexual notion of desire for the opposite sex, whether that was male or female. And while true that in non-medical literature, '[e]xtraordinary or "marvelous" events' in relation to sexual traits, were taken as 'possibilities inscribed in Nature [and] understood as manifestations of divine will' (Cleminson and Vázquez García, 2013, 7), the extent to which medical literature considered them atypical cases is called into question by at least one of the more popular and influential sources of the time, Juan Fragoso's *Cirvgia vniversal* (1581). Fragoso cited numerous examples of transformations of women into men, characterising them as events 'that happened naturally many times, both before and after birth, so as to fill the history texts, although some took it to be an exceptional occurrence'.[19] Still, the process that allowed for the possibility of phenomena like sex changes to be explained as relatively unremarkable, particularly in the case of women who transitioned into the more perfect form of men, then described as 'naturally' being attracted to women, simultaneously enabled the religious and social condemnation of homosexuality, decrying it as *contra natura*. 'In Castile and Spanish America', as the late María Elena Martínez reminded us, 'sodomy cases were mainly handled by the *audiencias* (royal tribunals) and church courts', with the 'overwhelming preponderance of men [being those] charged' (2016, 424, 425).

Following Aristotelian notions, most Spanish medical authors of the time subscribed to the idea that life began earlier for male fetuses than for female ones. Sources following Hippocrates's treatise *On the Nature of the Child* understood males to be formed at 30 days and females at 42. Hinojosos's timeline of 30 days for male fetuses coincides with this calculation as well

act directly. Lesbian desire is not explicitly acknowledged by Hinojosos, although it can be one way of reading Fragoso's remarks.

19 According to Fragoso, '[e]sto le aconteció muchas veces a [la] naturaleza, así estando la criatura en el vientre como de fuera: y de esto [es]tán llenas las historias, sino que algunos lo tuvieron por fabuloso' (1627, 162). The insistence in organising subjects along a male or female identity is evidenced in discussions on 'hermaphrodites'. For example, individuals 'possessing the natures of both sexes' were asked to 'choose one of these and swear before a bishop that they would remain true to this identity in order to ensure their heterosexuality for the rest of their lives' (Cleminson and Vázquez García, 2013, 49). Ambroise Paré (1510–90), one of the most well-known European surgeons of the time who classified different types of hermaphrodites, specified that those possessing 'both sets of organs well-formed' were obliged by law 'to choose which sex organ they wish to use, and they are forbidden on pain of death to use any but those they will have chosen, on account of the misfortunes that could result from such' (cited in Velasco, 2016, 100). Velasco points out that 'most cases of postnatal female-to-male transmutations were interpreted as success stories' reflecting the period bias which held on to Aristotelian notions of male perfection (2016, 100).

as with information in Damián Carbón's *Libro del arte delas Comadres, o madrinas* [Book on the art of midwives], which had been published in Mallorca in 1541, one of the texts to be printed in Spain in the sixteenth century focused specifically on women's medicine.[20] The *Libro del arte* declines to give an exact timeline on account of 'it being so well known that it is not necessary to determine it here [although] it is true that the general opinion is that the development of limbs is complete at thirty days at least, and at forty five days at most, and it is also far quicker if [the child] is male rather than female'.[21] Carbón's choice of language is tellingly misleading, given the relative unavailability of pregnant female cadavers in European medical circles; as Park explains, '[w]omen tended to die in or shortly after childbirth, rather than before it, which restricted the supply of bodies for private anatomy, and convicted criminals were rarely executed until after they had given birth' (2006, 188–89). This fact helps to explain Hinojosos's out-of-character statement to readers that he 'marvelled' at what he was able to observe inside the body of the pregnant woman, recalling that, in most other instances describing dissections (see chapter 2), he underscored just how unfazed he was by what he saw, with examinations of the inner body merely confirming what he professed he already knew to be true.

However, whereas Carbón accepted the Aristotelian idea that the place where the male seed was deposited helped to determine the sex of the child (the right side favoured males, the 'sinister' or left side, females), he offered no alternative sex categories. In his model, Hinojosos is likely drawing on Fragoso instead, an author he acknowledged elsewhere in the *Svmma*,[22] whose ideas also allowed for other possibilities along a sexual spectrum. In the *Cirvgia vniversal*, Fragoso had argued the following:

20 In addition to *the Libro del arte delas Comadres* there was a 1539 Salamantine edition of Paduan physician Paolo Bagellardo's *Opusculum recens natum de morbis puerorum* [Work on newborns and diseases in children]. Bagellardo's work, considered by many to be the first print source focused specifically on pediatrics, was published in different versions throughout Europe in the last quarter of the fifteenth century. There were also two texts that printed after Carbón's: Luis Lobera de Ávila's *Libro del regimiento de la salud, y de la esterilidad de los hombres y mugeres, y las muchas enfermedades de los niños* [Book on the regimen for good health, infertility in men and women, and many diseases in children], published in Valladolid in 1551; and Francisco Núñez's *El libro del parto humano* [Book on human childbirth], published in Alcala in 1580.

21 '[The time that passes since conception] está harto divulgado / y no es menester determinarlo aquí. Verdad es que la común opinión tiene / que la dicha hinchazón de miembros se cumple en treinta días lo más breve, y en cuarenta y cinco lo más largo, y también es más breve si es varón que si es hembra' (1541, fol. 15r).

22 Hinojosos mentions Fragoso by name in folios 142r and 149v of the 1595 edition of the *Svmma*. It is difficult to determine which edition of the *Cirvgia vniversal* he would have had access to given the dates, the one from 1581, 1586 or 1592; the first two were published in Madrid, the third in Alcala.

> Some claim that often nature has made a female, and she has been one in the mother's womb for some months, but having her genitals overcome by heat, they have been pushed out, and she has been turned into a man, which is then known through certain indecent movements they have toward men, and their voices are soft and melodious, and they are inclined toward women's work, and they fall into the nefarious sin, and on the contrary often nature has made a man with his genitals on the outside, and overcome by cold, they turn inwards, and he is made female. This is then known in [the person] having the airs and swagger of a man, as in her speech, and in all other movements and other things. ... From whence it is concluded that no man can be considered cold compared to women, nor a woman hot compared to a man.[23]

Like Vesalius and other anatomists of his day, Fragoso was increasingly concerned with observing unfolding processes in living specimens, not just anatomical structures in cadavers, which presented a practical problem that was partly resolved through the revival of animal vivisection; his knowledge of pregnancy, for instance, is informed by extensive experimentation on dogs.[24] Hinojosos's phrasing aligns the Hippocratic calculation of 30 days for the gendering of males extending it also to manly women, suggesting the possibility that his conclusion on fetuses becoming effeminate men at 60 days if heat rose by one degree would also be the case for the gendering of non-manly women, even though he neglects to include that fourth option.

As with the process of conception and sexual differentiation during early fetal development, the *Svmma*'s descriptions of pregnancy and childbirth are similar to what one finds in period European sources. Like Carbón, who explained that the colour of a woman pregnant with a male child was 'very light and pretty and ruddy' and her disposition 'light and not heavy and her appetite is not corrupt or bad, and her dreams are more delicious and delectable, the veins on her breasts are red and clearly visible, [and]

23 'muchas veces ha hecho naturaleza una hembra, y lo ha sido algunos meses en el vientre de su madre, y sobreviniendo a los miembros genitales copia de calor, salir afuera, y quedar hecho hombre, lo qual se conoce después en ciertos movimientos que tienen indecentes, para varones, tienen la voz blanda y melosa, son inclinados a hacer obras mujeriles, y caen en el pecado nefando, y por el contrario tiene muchas veces naturaleza hecho un varón con sus genitales afuera, y sobreviniendo frialdad se les vueluen adentro, y queda hecha hembra. Conócese después en tener el aire y meneos de varón, así [como] en la habla, como en todos los movimientos y otras. ... De donde colige que no hay hombre que se pueda llamar frío, respecto de la mujer, ni mujer caliente comparada al hombre' (1627, 162–63).

24 Whereas Fragoso's accounts of animal vivisection tend to focus on the movement of muscles and the flow substances, his description of the procedure of vivisecting pregnant dogs is uncharacteristically attentive to issues of motherhood and behaviour. For a discussion on the rise of animal testing in the early modern period, see Shotwell (2013).

her nipples are of a good colour',[25] Hinojosos likewise described a woman carrying a boy as displaying 'a healthy colour as before, and her right breast is larger than the left, and the breast is ruddy, and she feels the child on her right side, more pronounced, and she feels light on her feet'.[26] In contrast, if she was carrying a girl it was 'the opposite', and according to Hinojosos she '[has] spots on her face, and an ill complexion, and her skin is discoloured, and yellow, and the left breast is larger than the right, and its nipple black, and she feels uncomfortable, and has an appetite for unhealthy things'.[27]

However, when it comes to the possible outcomes of pregnancy, the *Svmma* differs from other European sources, attenuating a consideration of the monstrous in the context of the New World. As Sherry Velasco explains, '[w]hen considering the possibilities for narrating pregnancy, labor, and delivery in most medical, scientific, and certain popular texts we discover that they frequently resort to discussions of monsters to talk about descriptions of childbirth', and likewise 'early modern teratologies inevitably discuss the central role of mothers in the generation of monsters'.[28] Francisco Núñez, for example, in his *Libro del parto humano* [Book on human childbirth], published in Alcala in 1580, described the birth of 'a monster with horns, teeth and a tail', another case of a woman who had 'given birth to an elephant' and a slave who had done the same to 'a serpent'.[29] Carbón for his part claimed to have knowledge of a women who had given birth to 'an excess of twenty five chunks of meat resembling fish', and another who had delivered a male child inexplicably missing an arm until it was revealed that he had shared the womb with a creature 'shaped like a sea urchin' who had fed on his unfortunate companion during the gestation process.[30] Hinojosos, on the other hand, offers only one example of a monstrous birth in the phenomenon

25 'el color de la preñada es muy claro, lindo y colorado y más la disposición de la preñada es ligera y no pesada, y su apetito no es corrupto y malo, sus sueños son mas sabrosos y delectabes, en las tetas aparecen las venas coloradas y claras, los pezones de buen color' (1541, fol. 18v).

26 'si es hijo la mujer trae buena color como de antes, y tiene el pecho derecho mayor que el izquierdo, y el pecho bermejo, y siente el niño en el lado derecho, y más levantado, y se siente ligera para andar' (1595, fols. 170r–170v).

27 'al contrario si tiene la mujer paño en el rostro, o mala color, y está descolorida y amarilla, y el pecho izquierdo mayor que el derecho, y el pezón de él, negro, y mucho fastidio, y el apetito de cosas dañosas' (1595, fol. 170v).

28 Velasco refers to this phenomenon in early modern European sources as 'the monsterization of motherhood' (2016, 79).

29 In Núñez's words, 'un monstruo con cuernos y dientes y cola', 'una mujer llamada Alcippe [que] parió un elefante, y una esclava una serpiente' (1580, fols. 14v–15r).

30 'Vi en Mallorca la mujer de un oficial de aquella tierra parir un niño que le faltaba un brazo comido: y después de poco salir cierto animal semejante a erizo vivo y con dientes: tal que era maravilla ver tan espantable figura. También vi en dicha ciudad y lugar otra mujer parir más de veinte y cinco pedazos de carne de semejanza de peces' (1541, fol. 17r).

of the 'molomatrizes', which he describes as 'a tumour' resulting either from 'excessive cold in the seeds of the man as well as the woman', or from 'the seed of a woman being released by itself, without that of the man, and lacking heat at the moment of animation, it ceases to be a man and turns into a monster'.[31] Instead of an emphasis on the results of monstrous births as would be expected in sixteenth-century and early seventeenth-century Hispanic sources, the *Svmma* homes in on the female role in bringing about the molomatrizes, noting that it is women's 'pollution in dreams' [polución entre sueños], possibly referring to female masturbation and/or orgasm, that cause her seed to be released. The phenomenon is further gendered in a negative way by underscoring that 'these illnesses always befall women who have known men', by which a reader is to understand both 'married women and those who are not', subjects who share the common trait of no longer being virgins, regardless of whether they currently had a legal spouse or were having sex outside marriage; all are measured by the same standard.[32] Consequently, not only is the female sex drive vilified as potentially harmful to one's health in the text, but the figure of the sexually experienced woman is linked to monstrosity in ways that understand her body as unstable and unreliable. Women are thus again only partly at fault in their own health predicament, a position not unlike the one Cárdenas had argued a few years before in the case of dirt eaters in the *Problemas y secretos*.[33]

Like Hinojosos and Cárdenas, Agustín Farfán will offer his own discussion of many of the same topics as it relates to women's health. In the second edition of his *Tractado*, published just a year after the *Problemas y secretos* in 1592, the section on the links between problems in menstruation and women's unhealthy eating habits reads as if it were a gloss of Cárdenas's

31 'Molomatrizes, es un tumor, que se hace dentro de la madre ... las causas del molomatrizes son mucha frialdad en las simientes, así del varón, como de la mujer, y otras veces por derramarse la simiente de la mujer a solas, sin la del varón, y por faltarle calor al tiempo de animar, deja de ser hombre, y se hace monstruo' (1595, fol. 166v). While the *Svmma* will use the adjective monstruous to describe the negative effects of *caneros*, a type of wart that disfigured the mouth preventing patients from closing it or eating (1595, fol. 37v) and also in the case of varicose veins which could 'enlarge a leg to the size of a man's waist' (1595, fol. 71r), Hinojosos will use the noun 'monster' only twice in the book, in the two instances already cited. 'Engendro' is used only once, also in the section on *molomatrizes*.

32 'estas enfermedades siempre suceden a mujeres, que han conocido varón' (1595, fol. 166v); 'las casadas, que las que no lo son' (1595, fol. 167r).

33 There are contrasting views among scholars on whether entities that did not fit within the male and female sex categories were understood as monstrous during this period. For a discussion on hermaphrodites as 'praeter naturam' versus 'contra naturam' in the early modern context, extending to colonial Latin America, see in particular Cleminson and Vázquez García (2013), and Tortorici's 'Introduction: Unnatural Bodies, Desires and Devotions', 2016, 1–22, which also considers Hinojosos's 1595 edition of the *Svmma*.

work. 'These two things are done very well by the women of New Spain', declares Farfán,

> for at all hours of the day and many of the night you will see them eating treats. Mostly cocoa for eating or drinking, that they will not go without it. Others gorge themselves on chocolate, which is a drink made of thick things that do not agree with one another and are hard to digest. They eat green and unripe fruits all year long. Others cannot get enough limes with salt and bitter and sweet oranges. Others eat adobe soil and they do not leave a red jar uncovered, and even the jar itself that they do not swallow. And if this were done only by young women I would not be so shocked, but those who have their heads full of grey are more prone to vice and more undisciplined. These things thicken the blood, and constrict and obstruct the veins as if with rock and mud. And although I swear to them that it kills them (as they can see for themselves), they are not frightened, nor do the poor souls stop to consider that they commit a mortal sin. May God enlighten their understanding, so they do not find death at their own hands.[34]

At first glance, Farfán appears to be on the same page as Cárdenas in his opinions about women's unhealthy choices in the context of New Spain, with the same all-inclusive and totalising statements. However, physiological root causes are not mentioned in the *Tractado*. Women are chastised for behaving poorly and for placing their lives at risk, yet the path charted by Cárdenas and others delimiting their agency according to a substandard humoral constitution is considerably attenuated in Farfán's elaboration. He accepts that the breast milk produced by a woman if she is carrying a male child is more nutritious than if pregnant with a girl, explaining that sources more familiar with the subject so say ['como todos los que lo entienden lo afirman'] and that he finds no reason to contradict them ['que no hay para que tener opinión'], but it is as close as he will come to a position akin to that of his colleagues in New Spain (1592, 45v). Upon closer inspection,

34 'Estas dos cosas hacen muy bien las mujeres de la Nueva España, porque a todas horas del día y a muchas de la noche las verán comer golosinas. Mayormente el cacao comido y bebido, y éste no les ha de faltar. Otras se hartan de chocolate, que es una bebida hecha de muchas cosas entre sí muy contrarias, gruesas, y malas de digerir. Comen frutas verdes y mal maduras todo el año. Otras no se ven hartas de limas y sal y de naranjas agrias y dulces. Otras comen tierra de adobes, y no dejan tapadera de jarro colorado y aíun el jarro que no tragan. Y si esto que digo, hiciesen solas las mozas; no me espantara tanto, mas las que tienen las cabezas llenas de canas, son más viciosas, y más desregladas. Estas cosas engruesan la sangre, y opilan y tapan las venas, como con piedra y lodo. Y aunque les jure, que las mata (como ellas lo ven) no han [de] medrarse, ni reparan las pobres que pecan mortalmente. Alumbre Dios sus entendimientos, porque no tomen la muerte con sus manos' (1592, fols. 34v–34r).

and placed alongside other sections of the text that focus on women's health, a case can be made for the *Tractado* opening the door to women's empowerment in its rejection of a medicalised view that predetermines their weakness based on perceived anatomical or physiological shortcomings.[35]

Around 46 years old when the *Tractado* was first published, going by the portrait of the author included in the last folio of the first edition (see figure 3.1), Farfán claimed to have already been a practising doctor and surgeon for 27 years before deciding to write a book.[36] Citing a document suggesting he had supervised a medical student's examination at the University of Seville in the 1550s alongside Fuente, Somolinos believed him to be a graduate of that institution, although Farfán himself only discloses a link to the University of Alcala, suggesting the possibility he may have trained there instead (Somolinos, 1980a, 220; Farfán, 1579, 162v). He would go on to receive an American degree in 1567, proudly declaring himself 'a graduate of this illustrious University of Mexico' although, as Juan Comas notes, it is likely the degree was conferred by way of an exam rather than coursework given that the teaching of medicine had only just begun there at the time of the *Tractado*'s publication.[37] Based on a cross-comparison of archival documents, Somolinos concluded that Farfán had relatives in New Spain, which possibly motivated his decision to move there from Spain with his wife and daughter in 1557, going on to have two other children once he had settled overseas (1980a, 220–21). By 1568 he was a widower and decided to join the Augustinians, taking his vows a year later and changing his name from Pedro García to Agustín (Somolinos, 1980a, 222).

Although written in Spanish and, according to its author, in a 'clear and accessible style, so that anyone who wishes or has need [of surgery] can benefit from it',[38] both Bravo and Fuente pointed out to readers the erudite nature of the book in their respective endorsing signatures. In the first edition, Farfán seemed to embrace that characterisation, privileging a medical readership but allowing for the possibility that it would also benefit a non-expert public: it was a book for 'surgeons, those who practice surgery, those who need them, and those who lack them, and for doctors'.[39] The insistently repeated claim in the second, 1592 edition that it was a book 'for the people' rather than

35 For a fuller discussion on the link between Farfán's views on social interaction and relationships in New Spain and therapeutic innovation, see Pérez Marín (2020).

36 It should be noted that each of Farfán's editions was handled by a different printer: Antonio Ricardo in 1579; Pedro Ocharte in 1592; and Jerónimo Balli in 1610. The text of the 1610 edition follows closely the 1592 version, though the end result will be slightly shorter in the number of folios.

37 See Comas (1995, 108).

38 'modo de curar claro, e intelegible. Para que todos los que quisieren, y tuvieren necesidad, se aprovechen de ella' (1579, fol. 1r).

39 'los cirujanos, que ejercitan la cirugía, los que han menester, y los que carecieren de ellos, y de los médicos, se aprovechen de ella' (1579, fol. 1r).

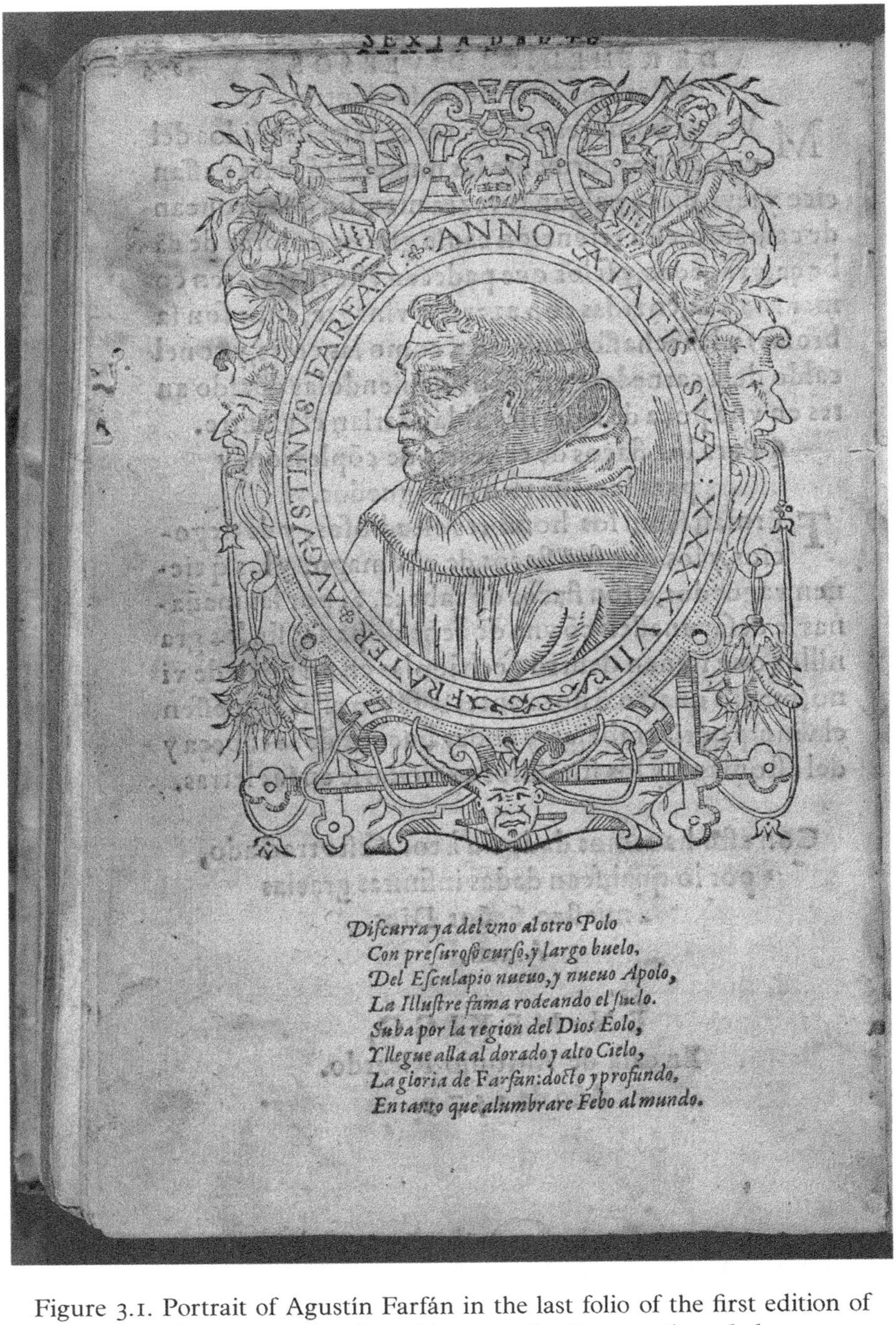

Figure 3.1. Portrait of Agustín Farfán in the last folio of the first edition of the *Tractado breve de anothomia y chirvgia, y de algvnas enfermedades, que mas comunmente suelen hauer en esta Nueua España* [Brief Treatise] (1579). Item 87097, courtesy of the Huntington Library, San Marino, California.

the medical establishment, was not as salient a consideration in 1579. The first version of the *Tractado* did have features that enhanced its accessibility beyond its choice of a romance language, namely a well-organised table of contents running the length of two full folios describing its six sections,[40] and an extremely detailed and lengthy alphabetised introductory table (at nine and a half folios) searchable by illness, remedy or body part. And yet, some sections took for granted a level of expertise that would have been beyond the reach of an untrained reader, as evidenced by an intriguing yet overlooked feature of the first edition, namely the presence of three small medical illustrations embedded within its prose content illustrating the placement of nerve tissue in one instance (see figure 3.2), and the shape of surgical incisions in the other two, images that are replaced with alphabetic characters and punctuation signs in subsequent printings.[41]

Yet despite its more specialised focus, there are signs already in the first version of an approach to medicine that would place greater emphasis than his contemporaries on narrative and on patients' subjectivity. In the section describing the cure for 'cancerous tumours' in both men and women, there is an extended passage on how to proceed when they are found in women's breasts.[42] Having surveyed Hippocrates and Galen, but claiming not to have found much of use in those sources other than a warning that the condition could lead to madness, Farfán turns instead to Lanfranc of Milan's[43] explanation for breast tumours. Lanfranc believed that the accumulation of blood that failed to turn into milk could become corrupted, generating the anomaly, with the onset of madness as secondary symptom rather than a root cause. The appropriate course of treatment was to take measures that reduced the inflammation, but Farfán cautions:

> I say that the things to be used to combat the inflammation should not be strong but light, and should be applied warm, such as rose oil, because strong ones steer the humour toward the heart, and because women's

40 The book is divided into: 1 – anatomy, 2 – abscesses, inflammation and tumors, 3 – tumors occurring specifically in the head, nose, mouth, testicles, breasts and joints, 4 – wounds, 5 – ulcers and 'bubas o mal francés', and 6 – stomach and intestinal problems.

41 For a detailed analysis of these images in the context of the intersection between cultural consolidation and the history of science in colonial Latin America, see Pérez Marín (2020). As mentioned in chapter 2, prior to Farfán, Bravo's *Opera medicinalia* (1570) had also featured images of a medical nature: an illustration of the veins in the thorax copied from Vesalius's *Venesection Letter* (1539), which incorrectly reversed the direction of the vena cava, as well as a botanical illustration of sarsaparilla.

42 Farfán gives several alternatives: 'cancro', 'çaratan', 'cancer' and 'caricinoma'.

43 Lanfranc of Milan had been a thirteenth-century physician who is credited with founding the French school of surgery, after he was exiled from Italy and relocated there.

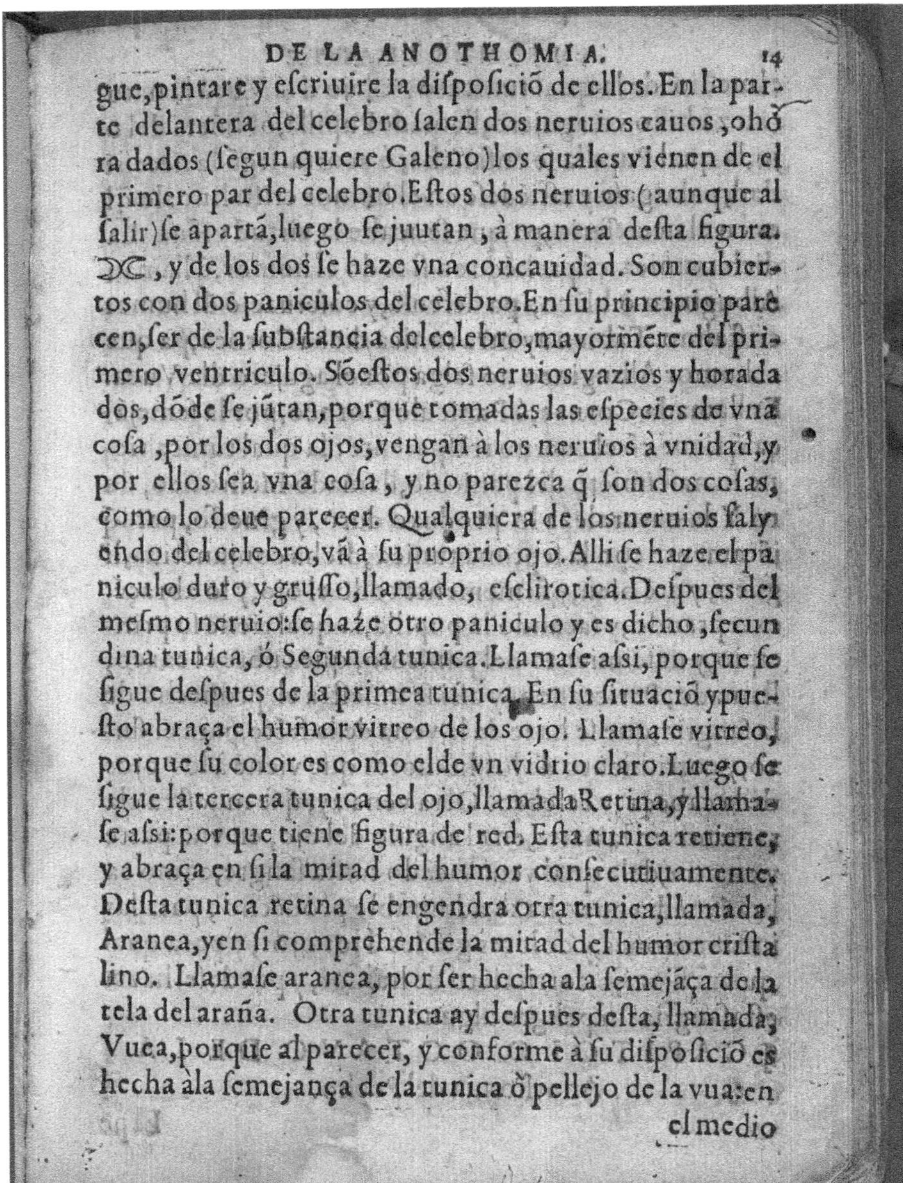

DE LA ANOTHOMIA. 14

gue, pintare y eſcriuire la diſpoſiciō de ellos. En la parte delantera del celebro ſalen dos neruios cauos, ohōrados (ſegun quiere Galeno) los quales vienen de el primero par del celebro. Eſtos dos neruios (aunque al ſalir) ſe apartā, luego ſe juntan, à manera deſta figura. ⊃⊂, y de los dos ſe haze vna concauidad. Son cubiertos con dos paniculos del celebro. En ſu principio parecen, ſer de la ſubſtancia del celebro, mayormēte del primero ventriculo. Son eſtos dos neruios vazios y horadados, dōde ſe jūtan, porque tomadas las eſpecies de vna coſa, por los dos ojos, vengan à los neruios à vnidad, y por ellos ſea vna coſa, y no parezca q̄ ſon dos coſas, como lo deue parecer. Qualquiera de los neruios ſalyendo del celebro, vā à ſu proprio ojo. Alli ſe haze el paniculo duro y gruſſo, llamado, eſclirotica. Deſpues del meſmo neruio: ſe haze otro paniculo y es dicho, ſecundina tunica, ó Segunda tunica. Llamaſe aſsi, porque ſe ſigue deſpues de la primea tunica. En ſu ſituaciō y pueſto abraça el humor vitreo de los ojo. Llamaſe vitreo, porque ſu color es como el de vn vidrio claro. Luego ſe ſigue la tercera tunica del ojo, llamada Retina, y llamaſe aſsi: porque tiene figura de red. Eſta tunica retiene, y abraça en ſi la mitad del humor conſecutiuamente. Deſta tunica retina ſe engendra otra tunica, llamada, Aranea, y en ſi comprehende la mitad del humor criſtalino. Llamaſe aranea, por ſer hecha ala ſemejāça de la tela del araña. Otra tunica ay deſpues deſta, llamada, Vuea, porque al parecer, y conforme à ſu diſpoſiciō es hecha àla ſemejança de la tunica ō pellejo de la vua: en

el medio

Figure 3.2. Folio 14r of the 1579 edition of Agustín Farfán's *Tractado* showing a small medical image resembling half moons embedded in the text as part of an anatomical description. The passage explains how the two nerves connecting the brain to the eyes separate and then meet again 'a manera de esta figura' ['in the manner shown in this figure']. Item 87097, courtesy of the Huntington Library, San Marino, California.

> breasts (in feeling pain) are comparable to men's testicles: for this reason we shall take every available measure to mitigate the pain.[44]

Farfán engages in the uncommon gesture in medical literature of the time of inviting a male surgeon or doctor reading his text to consider a situation from a female point of view, particularly in regard to experiences of discomfort and pain. Compared to both Benavides and Hinojosos, Farfán devotes far more textual space to the interaction he has with patients: at the moment of diagnosis, when listing alternative forms of treatment for those who had limited access to medicines by virtue of where they lived, or when describing follow-up care, the latter not typical of medieval surgical exempla where the quick confirmation of a positive outcome was usually the end of a given case study.

The original 1579 version of the *Tractado* had been a quarto in 8s edition of 274 folios; the 1592 version was roughly 20 per cent longer, also a quarto in 8s edition but comprised of 353 folios. Farfán himself pointed out the differences between the two to readers in his preface; the second book went well beyond a mere reprinting, and was 'reformed and expanded, new in almost everything'.[45] The introductory table was shortened and moved to the end, and the contents of the first text were redistributed into five sections, each one identified as its own treatise. If we put Farfán's claim to the test we find that the section on anatomy, which had gone first in the 1579 edition, was placed last in the 1592 version without significant changes otherwise. However, the rest of the material was indeed revised and expanded, albeit in a less straightforward manner. Treatises 1 and 2 in the second printing both dealt with medicine more generally, discussing topics that ranged from pain management, to *bubas* to irregularities in menstruation; the third chapter dealt with fevers; the fourth, with the treatment of wounds all seemingly covering the same ground as before. It is only upon a close reading that the increased presence of women as subject matter is uncovered, for unlike the case of Hinojosos's second *Svmma* where the headings of the new sections called attention to paediatrics and obstetrics, in the second edition of Farfán's *Tractado*, women were instead integrated into discussions on New World health rather than treated in isolation.

Compared to how the human body was described in Hispanic medical sources of the period, the bodily template scrutinised by Farfán lends itself far more easily to being read as female. The *Tractado*, particularly in its second edition, is peppered with references to female patients, and contains

44 'digo que las cosas que se han de poner para reprimir la Inflamación, no sean fuertes sino leves, y se han de poner tibias, así como aceite rosado, porque las fuertes hacen ir el humor al corazón, y porque las tetas de las mujeres (en el sentir del dolor) son comparadas a los testículos de los hombres; por esta razón habemos de poner toda la solicitud y cuidado, en mitigar el dolor' (1579, fol. 180v).

45 'aunque otra vez impresa, sale la segunda [edición] reformada y añadida, que es casi de nuevo en todo' (1592, unnumbered verso folio preceding fol. 1r).

special instructions to accommodate their needs. Instead of individual cases, the chapters are often presented as first-person reflections on how patients reacted to different medical treatments. It is in this manner that women enter the text, not as dissected specimens as in Hinojosos's work, or as individual case studies, but as a chorus of female voices conversing with him. And by the second edition, he has quite a bit to say about women, and they to him.

Chocolate drinkers and mud eaters were not Farfán's only unruly female patients. Others who sought out his help included women who suffered from chronic headaches because they insisted on changing the colour of their hair:

> All of these pains and greater ones are endured by the women who dye their hair blonde, having their heads wet for weeks on end with lye and mud, and other concoctions that they make. And in exchange for looking fine for one day, and pray to God that they do not look worse in the eyes of their Creator, they want to suffer all their lives excessive pains. If they call the doctor they then want him upon arrival to relieve them of their pain in one hour. And they do not realise that more time is needed to treat the problem, which they have endured for many years.[46]

Texts on women's medicine like the *Trotula* tended to include cosmetic remedies to treat skin conditions or to colour hair, which may explain why these topics surface as subject matter in the 1592 *Tractado* in the first place if Farfán is consulting existing medical treatises on women's medicine to develop his own work. But what is distinctive about his idiosyncratic approach is that when it comes to procedures like lightening the skin or the hair, rather than framing the discussion as a supplement to expert advice from other medical sources and his own practice, as he does for matters pertaining to fertility and childbirth, he uses these moments instead to put forth humorous critiques that poke fun at women's stubborn ways.[47] The

46 'Todos estos dolores y mayores padecen las mujeres que se enrubian, trayendo toda la semana las cabezas mojadas con lejías y barros, y otros badulaques, que ellas hacen. Y a trueco de parecer bien un día, y plega a Dios que no parezcan más mal, a los ojos de su creador, quieren padecer toda su vida excesivos dolores. Si llaman al médico, quieren, que en llegando les quite el dolor en una hora. Y no reparan, que es menester más tiempo, para curarlas del mal, que ha que padecen muchos años' (1592, fol. 123r).

47 Inca Garcilaso de la Vega echoes Farfán in his own description of hair dyeing practices in the *Comentarios reales* [Royal Commentaries] (1609), describing the 'voluntary torment' [tormento voluntario] endured by women in Peru who dyed their hair black. Although shocking to him as a boy, once in Spain, Inca Garcilaso remarks he was 'no longer surprised, seeing what many ladies do to lighten their hair, that they douse it in sulfur and soak it in etching acid and put it out in the sun at midday … that I do not know which is worse for good health, if this [Spanish women dyeing their hair blonde] or that [Andean women dyeing their hair black] … Of all this and much more is capable the pursuit of beauty' ['Pero en España he perdido la admiración, viendo lo que muchas damas hacen para enrubiar sus cabellos, que

female chorus in the *Tractado* is seldom compliant and comes across as a group of demanding consumers. Women experiencing the menopause, for whom Farfán recommends a strict regimen excluding most fruits and vegetables but amenable to raisins, green and dry figs, cooked chicory, asparagus, capers with parsley and black garbanzo bean broth, react unreasonably to his spartan dietary advice, he complains:

> When menstruation stops completely, that does no more than signal the month with one or two drops of blood, and with pain in the hips, some women become yellowish, others purplish, others pale as if deceased. They lose their appetite and, like pregnant women, they go about eating in secret, hiding in corners, which harms them. They cannot walk two steps that they are not out of breath from being swollen like dropsy sufferers. When told to show greater discipline they become cross and angry, as if you have insulted them.[48]

Both patients' and doctor's reactions and emotions make it onto the page. 'There is so much variation in the natural course of many women's menses that I am shocked',[49] writes Farfán in the first lines of his long section on women's menstruation, one of the longest in the body of the second edition as a whole. There is a familiar cadence to how Farfán narrates the episodes just cited which is reminiscent of the medieval *fablieux*. Women in their folly pay no heed to the wise counsel Farfán gives them, despite his best intentions, leading him to ask the reader to share in his frustration at being unable to persuade them. To an extent the text can be seen as a New World manifestation of what Encarnación Juárez-Almendros calls 'the aggressive literary treatment' of the trope of the ageing woman in early modern Hispanic literature, where marginal female figures [are] often portrayed as a hag or a witch, and like the prostitute 'embody and symbolize patriarchal beliefs relating to female imperfection', made to 'display the extreme consequences of uncontrollable bodies' (2017, 11). 'In contrast with the cultural representation of old men', underscores Juárez-Almendros, 'which mostly emphasizes attributes of wisdom and dignity, descriptions of old women [in early modern Spanish literature] center on their corporeal decay and moral depravity'

los perfuman con azufre y los mojan con agua fuerte de dorar y los ponen al sol en medio del día ... que no sé cuál es peor y más dañoso para salud, si esto o aquello ... Tanto como esto y mucho más puede el deseo de la hermosura'] (2003, 590).

48 'Cuando la regla falta del todo, que no hace más, de señalar el mes con una o dos gotas de sangre, y con dolores de las caderas, andan algunas mujeres amarillas, otras como moradas, y blanquecinas, y como difuntas. Quítaseles la gana de comer, y como mujeres preñadas andan por los rincones comiendo a hurtadillas, lo que les daña. No pueden andar dos pasos que luego no se ahogen, de hinchadas como hidrópicos. Diciéndoles que se rijan bien se enojan y aíran, como afrentadas' (1592, fols. 40r–40v).

49 'Es tan diferente el bajar la regla naturalmente en muchas mujeres, que a mí me espanta' (1592, fol. 33r).

(2017, 85). But unlike fictional and theatrical examples of this characterisation, there is a darker undertone to Farfán's appropriation in the context of a medical text, for despite women's temporary triumph in asserting their agency and demanding a degree of control over their bodies that defies an expert opinion, within the medical and scientific universe of the work, they do so at great cost, putting their lives in danger. The *Tractado*, therefore, never ends a chapter on these moments of comic relief, but goes on to provide instructions for remedies and various forms of treatment. The incorporation of literary models enlivens the text but does not compromise its didactic function, doing the work of both science and literature, and arguably communicating with a reader of the period more effectively because of that interplay. After all, it is Farfán's *Tractado* that will run into the highest number of editions for a medical text, more than any other title from early colonial Mexico and an unusual feat when compared to locally printed sixteenth century books on secular subject matter, regardless of their choice of topic. The book's editorial success would suggest that Farfán's writing satisfied the expectations of his New World reading public.[50]

The horizon of female characters in the *Tractado* creates a gendered straw man adversary for Farfán that enables him to debunk erroneous medical ideas in arguments likely aimed at a wider readership, including other male medical practitioners. It is a process similar to the hypothetical questions used by Cárdenas in the context of *problemata* so as to justify including information elucidating a given subject. The conceit of a female chorus, for example, provides the narrative frame for his discussion of stomach problems believed to be caused by the collapsing of the 'paletilla' [the xiphisternum],[51] and is the central prompt of the section of the text dealing with pain in the womb. Farfán writes:

50 Five copies are known to survive of the 1592 edition, held at the Biblioteca Museo del Hombre, the Huntington Library, the John Carter Brown Library, the Biblioteca Palafoxiana and the Benson Collection at the University of Texas, Austin. A facsimile edition of this version was published by Ediciones Cultura Hispánica in Madrid in 1944, although it is unclear which copy was used or if marginalia was suppressed. The copy at the Palafoxiana has been digitised and is available online via the Primeros Libros de las Américas portal. Although beyond the scope of this study, we note that there are several surviving copies of the 1610 edition of the *Tractado*, for example, at the Benson Collection, at Yale University's Medical Historical Library, at the US National Library of Medicine and the Wellcome Library.

51 'Cosa común es decir las mujeres que se cae la paletilla del estómago, siendo imposible, por ser un hueso muy pegado a su compañero' (1592, fol. 154v). The xiphisternum is a structure made of cartilage attached to the lower part of the sternum that can become detached. However, from a modern anatomical lens, Farfán would be correct in ascertaining that it could not be restored to its original position with the treatment he claims is followed by women. The belief in the 'caída de la paletilla' seems to be of European origin and is still discussed today in the context of South American traditional medicine. See Rodríguez López (1910, 106).

> Women who say their wombs become suffocated and rise to their stomachs are completely mistaken because it cannot rise that far, as it has very strong ligaments and nerves that do not give it that [much] space [to move]; that it would shift toward one side of the body or another, or go lower a bit, yes, but for it to rise is impossible … What seems like suffocation is gas that presses against the diaphragm when it rises, it being a very necessary and essential instrument for breathing, and all of you women believe me that this is the truth.[52]

Seemingly addressing female readers directly and unequivocally—'créanme todas' [all of you women, believe me] as opposed to 'todos'—, the author's remarks still target a broader audience that adhered to the Greco-Roman idea of the wandering womb. According to Plato in the *Timaeus*, the womb was a separate organism within women, 'an animal desirous of procreating children' which, if left unfertilised beyond youth, would 'suffer the restraint with difficulty … wandering every way through the body, obstruct[ing] the passage of breath … and caus[ing] all-various diseases' (1955, 222). So-called '*furor uterinus*', as Laurinda Dixon explains, could be treated by 'fumigating the vagina with sweet-smelling vapors … or, conversely, inhaling foul-smelling substances … to repel the organ and drive it from the upper parts of the body' (1995, 16). Despite the fact that the notion of the wandering womb had been superseded in learned medical circles in most of Europe by the sixteenth century, remedies used to treat female ailments well into the seventeenth century often included attract/repel methods involving vaginal fumigation, even if the original rationale for the procedure no longer registered. The chorus of women resisting Farfán's advice, therefore, should not be seen necessarily as ignorant folk merely relying on their physical sensations to draw novel conclusions, expressing instead an embodied experience of older, once authorised, medical knowledge.

Likewise, exploring the subject of women allows Farfán to venture into topics that would have been difficult to air in a more standard forum like a medical compendium, such as aphrodisiacs to enhance a man's sexual performance, especially considering his station as an Augustinian friar, notwithstanding his previous experience as a married man. The justification for addressing the issue in the *Tractado* will be the question of happiness within marriage: 'God created man and gave him woman as a companion and gift, forming her from the very rib of man so that he would better love and

52 'Engáñanse en todo, las mujeres, que dicen, las ahoga la madre, porque se les sube al estómago. Y aunque les parece a ellas así no puede subir tanto, porque tiene muy fuertes ligaduras de cuerdas, y nervios, que no le darán ese lugar, encogerse hacia un lado y otro del cuerpo, y bajarse un poco, esto só; mas subir es imposible … Lo que parece que ahoga, son ventosidades, que subiendo arriba, comprimen y aprietan el diafragme, que es un instrumento muy necesario, y forzoso, para la respiración, y créanme todas, que ésta es la verdad' (1592, fol. 72v).

care for her', writes Farfán; he 'joined them and married them' so that 'man (moved by the desire of the flesh) would not sin'.[53] Infertility compromised the stability of a couple's relationship for 'married men (when they do not have children) are not happy, and it seems that they do not love their wives. And then when God grants them to him, the passions and the quarrels cease with such great tokens of love, as are children.'[54] For that reason, the author explains that he was:

> moved by Christian charity to give remedy to some poor men who live very sad and disappointed with their wives. Because although healthy and young, and with some vigour and will, [they] have such small penises that come the natural act, they lose their energy in such a way as if they were not men. If this remedy were not good for having children, it will be good for paying the conjugal debt, which they have as an obligation. And thus with it they will cease to cause much offense to Our Lord, and let Him (on account of who He is) not allow that this remedy be used by some soulless men who would offend Him, that this is not my intention, but rather what I have said above.[55]

Farfán treads on dangerous ground, recognising that his advice may be put to use by men outside a marital context, invoking God's omnipotence as a shield against the prospect that the information he has shared might be misused. Even if the remedies listed do not have an immediate effect, he continues, sexual therapy should be attempted for a period of 'one or two months', at which point his male reader should act thus: 'feeling within you more vigour and strength, commit yourself to God, so that with His favour you will achieve His holy wish'.[56] Farfán's tone is casual but careful, self-consciously

53 'Dios crió al hombre [y] le dio por compañera y regalo a la mujer, y formóla de una de las costillas del mismo hombre para que más la amase, y quisiese. Juntólos Dios y casólos porque el género humano se aumentase y creciese, y porque el hombre (instigado y movido con la concupiscencia de la carne) no pecase' (1592, fols. 230v–231r).

54 'los hombres casados (cuando no tienen hijos) no andan contentos, y parece que no quieren bien a sus mujeres. Y cuando Dios se los da entonces cesan las pasiones y las rencillas con tan grandes prendas de amor, como son los hijos' (1592, fol. 231r).

55 'lo que me movió y obliga con caridad cristiana a dar remedio a algunos pobres, que viven muy tristes y desgustados con sus mujeres. Los cuales aunque tienen salud, y son de edad juvenil, y aunque tienen alguna potencia y voluntad, tienen tan flacos los miembros genitales, que en llegando al acto natural, aflojan de tal manara, como si no fuesen hombres. Cuando este remedio no aprovechase, para tener hijos, aprovechará para pagar el débito que deben de obligación. Y así con él se dejarán de hacer muchas ofensas a nuestro Señor, y él (por quien es) no permita se aprovechen de este remedio algunos desalmados, para ofenderle, que no es tal mi intento, sino el que arriba dejo dicho' (1592, fols. 231r–231v).

56 'Usen de este remedio un mes, o dos, y cuando sientan en sí más potencia y fuerza, encomiéndese a Dios, que con su favor conseguirá su santo deseo' (1592, fol. 233v).

humorous as in other passages of the text but never mocking on account of a person's medical condition. A patient's stubbornness or attitude may be derided but not his or her physical limitations or state of mind when related to physiological processes.

Arguably the more transgressive element in the passage is the opinion that his medical advice should be followed even 'if this remedy were not good for having children', volunteering an unusual reading of the notion of marital debt under canon law. The 'dissolution of a marriage on the grounds of frigidity or impotence', as Sara McDougall explains, was a solution more often sought by women than by men, at least in Europe, despite the fact that within marriages, it also 'functioned to allow men to have sex with their wives on demand, but not the reverse' (2013, 175, 170). The raison d'être of the marital debt was the expectation that children would be produced in a Church-sanctified union so as to follow the Lord's command in Genesis 1:28 to 'Be fruitful and multiply, and replenish the earth'. But Farfán's recommendation of a treatment allowing for the possibility of sex that did not result in conception, as well as his emphasis on how the activity improves a couple's relationship, airs an uncommon point of view compared to how the matter was usually discussed in period sources that mentioned conjugal sexual intercourse. His was a remedy for happiness and for the social stability of New World societies as much as it was a medical treatment for a health problem.

The *Tractado* sits on the fence when it comes to the issue of power dynamics between men and women in sexual relationships, containing information that could be used either to empower women or to increase their submission. Despite a phrasing that would acknowledge a woman's will in the chapter on 'having children, for women who wish to do so' [Para que paran, las que lo desean], it is easy to see how a woman could feel coerced into a pregnancy if a third party attempted to make use of the medical advice to that end. And yet, supporting the view that the *Tractado* would have been less amenable to that interpretation is what Farfán chooses *not* to include if we compare his text to those by Hinojosos, Carbón and others that discussed pregnancy. Farfán, father to at least one daughter, recommends no special procedures for gender selection to ensure the procreation of boys rather than girls. Gone also are allusions to Hippocratic medicine that negatively marked the bodies of women carrying a female fetus but beautified those who were pregnant with a male child, despite his concession on the difference in the quality of breast milk cited earlier. His selective glossing of elements from these types of sources takes them in a new direction, also editing information hitherto relevant only to women, particularly on matters of cosmetics, and extending it so as to apply to men as well.[57] Discussions that in women's

57 For a discussion on some examples of Iberian period sources denouncing men's interest in cosmetic matters as unseemly, see Cabré (2011, 187–88).

health manuals concerned only their skin become in the *Tractado* remedies for 'the spots or pimples that afflict the faces of women *and men*' (emphasis added).[58] Farfán anticipates criticism on this point from readers who would have noticed the departure from the norm, pre-emptively answering them in his chapter on facial wounds: 'To he who says that I use medicines that are too fancy in these treatments I say that nothing is too good as far as the face is concerned, since it adorns and increases the good appearance of the man'; likewise, when suturing, 'the stitches joining the flesh and the skin should be very small and evenly spaced, leaving less of a mark'.[59] He cautions men who, after receiving facial injuries, sought out what today would be deemed plastic or cosmetic surgery: 'In the case of unseemly facial scars, some have tried to remove them, promising those who have them that they will make them more handsome and they will not be left so ugly'; however, writes Farfán, 'I have yet to see them deliver what they promise, for instead they leave the poor souls uglier and worse for wear. And thus I advise surgeons to not attempt these things, and to the patient, to not consent to them.'[60]

'Leaving behind, thus, questions on medicine',[61] as Farfán himself admits, in the *Tractado* period readers found a work that ceded a considerable amount of textual space to a portrait of their society as they then saw it. Farfán addressed his readers as patients and as selective consumers of medical services and remedies, but also from a platform that largely assumed a position of shared racial privilege, fellow members of New Spain's incipient colonial social fabric invested in representations of themselves as fundamentally European rather than partly (or fully) Indigenous or African. On this point, Farfán, and likely a large proportion of his audience, were on the same page, unconcerned with what are to us glaring omissions compromising our ability as scholars to better understand the full spectrum of subjective and embodied points of view that existed in the early modern period. And yet, despite these insurmountable obstacles to performing intersectional readings addressing questions on race and ethnicity and how they may have affected

58 'Para unos barros o espinas que nacen en el rostro a las mujeres y a los hombres' (1592, fol. 135v).

59 'Al que dijere, que pongo en esta cura mediçinas esquisitas, respondo, que todo lo merece la cara, pues hermosea y adorna al hombre. … Dije que diesen los puntos menudos, porque la carne y los cueros se juntan, e igualan mejor, y queda menos señal' (1592, fol. 298v).

60 'Algunos han querido (cuando las señales de la cara queda{n} fea{s}) quitarla(s), prometiendo a los que las tienen, de que los hermosearán, y les harán que no queden feos. Y hasta hoy he visto que hayan hecho lo que prometen, mas antes han dejado a los pobres más feos, y más puestos del lodo. Y así aconsejo al cirujano, que no se ponga en estas cosas, y al paciente, que no lo consienta' (1579, fol. 158v). For a discussion on how facial scars could affect social mobility in ways that apply to an early modern context, see Porter (2005) and Skinner (2015).

61 'Dejando pues cuestiones de medicina, porque no escribo (como he dicho otras veces) para médicos' (1595, fol. 33v).

the kinds of relationships readers forged with the *Tractado*, because for Farfán at least female patients' needs were an important consideration, his book still emerges as an unlikely safe haven that preserves a partial view of women's voices, albeit skewed toward those of European descent, displaying evidence of their critical discernment often altogether lost in period historiographical materials.

Not entirely against the tide but more holding its place within a wave of scholarly interventions witnessing a progressive increase in the medicalisation of gender difference, Farfán's treatment of women's health is a historical cul-de-sac. It would be popular with the readers of the time whose interest seems to have justified the *Tractado*'s multiple printings, and it possibly reached a comparatively larger number of female readers than would medical books of later eras, as the gulf between women's education and sites of new scientific knowledge-production only widened through their institutionalised exclusion from places of higher learning. However, in the end, Farfán's more relatable, community-embedded approach to writing on health topics did not blaze a new trail. Anatomy proved an unreliable ally to the medical establishment over the next centuries when it came to unearthing conclusive evidence of difference related to gender and race. Instead, the sustained interest in physiology, lasting all the way to the dawn of the twentieth century, and already reflected in the work of authors like Hinojosos and Cárdenas, helped to support the means by which science would throw its weight behind constructs of patriarchal social stratification, in colonial Latin America as it did elsewhere.

CHAPTER 4

Contested medical knowledge and regional self-fashioning

The first sentences of Juan de Cárdenas's *Primera parte de los problemas y secretos marauillosos de las Indias* [First part of the problems and marvellous secrets of the Indies] (1591) describe the Indies[1] as a land of boundless and wondrous natural resources, rich in every respect, but one:

> Asia, Africa and Europe need not complain, for they have and have had more writers to write about them than things to be written about. What could Pliny say or convey of the crocodile that the local [*indiano*] philosopher does not write of the caiman of this land? For if its properties are compared with those of the crocodile, those of the caiman are more notable and excellent. ... What did Avicenna say of turtles that there is not much more [to be said about] our turtles [*indianas icoteas*][2] for the shells of some are so large that they usually can hold six men. What do the authors write about the lizard that we are not able to say in the Indies about iguanas? What did Dioscorides write about the sea urchin that does not pale in comparison with the properties of the armadillo of New

1 Like other humanists of his time, Cárdenas used the term 'Indies' to denote America, the Philippines, and coastal areas in the Far East, the latter seen as distinct from Asia.

2 Today the name *icoteas* refers to *Trachemys scripta*, but Cárdenas may have had in mind a different species, as these do not grow to be very large. He was possibly referring to the Galápagos tortoise (*Chelonoidis nigra*). The islands had been discovered by Fray Tomás de Berlanga in 1535 and were featured in Abraham Ortelius's 1570 world map, the *Theatrum Orbis Terrarum* (see Figueras Vallés's 2010 study *Fray Tomás de Berlanga. Una vida dedicada a la Fe y la Ciencia*). Berlanga's account to Charles V mentioned tortoises, iguanas and he personally brought to Spain a caiman whose desiccated carcass has survived and is still a popular display with tourists who visit the Colegiata de Santa María del Mercado in Berlanga de Duero, Soria. Given the order of elements in Cárdenas's text, it is likely he had Berlanga's descriptions in mind. Another contender given the information he would have had access to at the time of the *Secretos*'s composition is the giant South American river turtle (*Podocnemis expansa*).

Spain? … Thus, herbs, fruits, fish and animals, what books would suffice to describe them all?[3]

Along with writers like Francisco Cervantes de Salazar (1514–75) and Bernardo de Balbuena (1568–1627), descriptions such as this one place Cárdenas in the company of some of the strongest apologists of New Spain in the early colonial period, as he makes a case for the value of both its natural resources and of the small but thriving society that had arisen there in the wake of the restructuring of Tenochtitlan into Mexico City (see figure 4.1a).[4] The opening section of his book is laden with imagery reminiscent of the initial Columbian gesture that had coded the islands of the Caribbean into a prelapsarian paradise. But in his version written almost a century later, the similes linking the two spaces have been replaced by competitive analogies where the New World is at least the Old's equal and, in some respects, it has the edge. The natural environs of the Indies are no longer 'green and beautiful like those of Spain in May', as Columbus had volunteered in the 'Letter to Santángel'.[5] Instead, for Cárdenas the resemblances underscored how what lay in the Americas was not necessarily superior in the sense of being more healthful or of better quality, but it was certainly more interesting from an epistemological standpoint, holding the promise of revealing new information in ways the 'known world' could not. If we read closely, his opening remarks are not directly about the flora and fauna of the Indies or its mineral wealth but rather about their textual representations, the untapped potential for that part of the world to generate knowledge compared to places that had already been described and studied: 'all of this land can rightfully lament that, despite its excess of subject matter, and abundance of strange, excellent and great things, it lacks those who would let them be known and bring them to light', reads the text.[6] Abundance is

3 'No tendrá Asia, África y Europa que quejarse, pues tiene y ha tenido más escritores que de ellas escriban, que cosas que poderse escribir. ¿Qué pudo decir ni encarecer Plinio del cocodrilo, pues no escriba el filósopho indiano del caimán de esta tierra? Pues cotejadas sus propiedades con las del cocodrilo, son las del caimán muy notables y excelentes. … ¿Qué dijo Avicenna de las tortugas que no haya mucho más en nuestras indianas icoteas, pues hay algunas en cuya concha suelen caber casi seis hombres? ¿Qué escriben los autores del lagarto, que no digamos en las Indias de las iguanas? ¿Qué escribió Dioscórides del erizo, que no se oscurezca con las propiedades del armadillo de la Nueva España?. … Pues yerbas, frutas, pescados y animales, ¿qué libros serían bastantes para poderlo todo poner en suma?' (1591, fols. 2r–3r).

4 For an in-depth study of the degree to which colonial urban planning in Mexico City at the time still relied heavily on the technologies and structures of the former Mexica state, see Mundy, *The Death of Aztec Tenochtitlan, the Life of Mexico City* (2015).

5 The trees of Hispaniola are 'tan verdes y hermosos como son por mayo en España' (1995, 221).

6 'vuelvo a decir que se puede con justa razón lamentar toda esta indiana tierra, de que sobrándole materia, y copia de extrañas, y excelentes grandezas, le falta quien las predique, y saque a luz' (1591, fol. 2r).

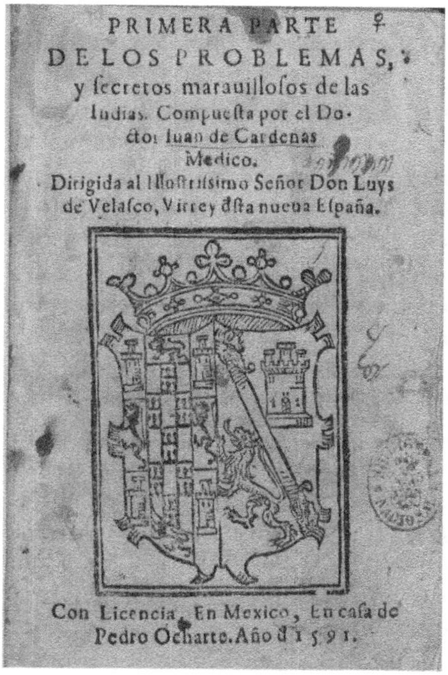

PRIMERA PARTE
DE LOS PROBLEMAS,
y ſecretos marauilloſos de las
Indias. Compueſta por el Do-
ctor Iuan de Cardenas
Medico.
Dirigida al Illuſtriſsimo Señor Don Luys
de Velaſco, Virrey deſta nueua Eſpaña.
Con Licencia, En Mexico, En caſa de
Pedro Ocharte. Año de 1591.

NVEVA
FILOSOFIA
DELA NATVRALEZA
del hombre, no conocida ni alcançada
de los grandes filoſofos antiguos: la
qual mejora la vida y ſalud humana. Com-
pueſta por doña Oliua Sabuco.
Con priuilegio,
En Madrid, por P. Madrigal.
M. D. LXXXVII.

Figures 4.1a and 4.1b. On the left, the title page of the 1591 edition of Juan de Cárdenas's *Primera parte de los problemas y secretos marauillosos de las Indias* [Problems and marvellous secrets of the Indies]. On the right, the title page of Oliva Sabuco de Nantes Barrera's *Nveva filosofia dela natvraleza del hombre* [The new philosophy of human nature] (1587). Courtesy of the Biblioteca Nacional de España.

showcased but only to underline what Cárdenas sees as the region's extreme scarcity: 'I have said all this', he writes, bringing the section to a close, 'so that the misery of this land may be properly understood, lacking only writers to illustrate and celebrate its things.'[7] For all its riches, the New World was poor without a lettered culture of its own.

To the modern reader, Cárdenas's navel-gazing is as chilling as it is emblematic. The various peoples that inhabited the Americas had a long-standing engagement with artistic and cultural representation, and had developed different forms of literacy by the time these words were being printed in 1591. Andean khipus of llama and vicuña fibres used in textual performances, Arawak petroglyphs and *areitos* re-enacting myths and oral history, Mayan script, which recorded syllabic characters and logograms

7 'He dicho todo esto ... para que con razón se entienda la lástima de esta tierra, pues a ella solo [le] faltaron escritores que ilustrasen y engrandeciesen sus cosas' (1591, fol. 3r).

on amatl and stone, all these are made to vanish in the *Problemas y secretos* in one fell swoop. In the geographic area closest to the author, by the time of Cortés's arrival, the member city-states of the Triple Alliance (the Aztec capital, Texcoco and Tlacopan) as well as the surrounding entities that resisted them (Tlaxcala, Otompan and Chalca) shared traditions of performative lyric poetry. Likewise, some Indigenous forms of representation not only survived but thrived after the fall of Tenochtitlan, incorporated into collaborative, European-guided projects like the Badianus Codex (see chapter 1) or Fray Bernardino de Sahagún's Florentine Codex (begun circa 1529 and completed in 1579), or in a more independent fashioning, continuing and even expanding, as in the case of artistic practices like *amantecayotl* [feather art] which, as Alessandra Russo notes, citing Sahagún, were 'everywhere in this New Spain' (2010, 12). If the bonfires of codices and cultural treasures held across the region in the mid sixteenth century had burned so bright that these objects sometimes forced themselves back into being by way of the European representations that told of their destruction,[8] Cárdenas's prose would write them out of existence altogether. The 'fantasy of emptiness', as Daniel Nemser calls it, became 'the condition' for the organisation of colonial space, and understood any and all forms of pre-Hispanic representation, from monumental culture and large-scale urban planning to intangible cultural heritage, as residual rather than foundational (2017, 32).[9] Colonial-era prose, like the maps that paved the way for the physical restructuring of colonial space, used paper in order to clear a path for initiatives that would bring to fruition what was, from a Eurocentric perspective, the land's true potential.

Although largely forgotten by the second half of the seventeenth century, if we compare the readings of the *Problemas y secretos* that took place within the first decades after its publication against those that the work generated in the twentieth century, the exercise brings into sharper focus Cárdenas's place within a genealogy of colonial discourse. Published a second time in 1913 by Mexico's then newly restructured National Museum of Archaeology, History and Ethnography [Museo Nacional de Arqueología, Historia y Etnografía], it would not be until the late 1950s and early 1960s that the

8 One of the more notorious examples is the 'Burning of the idols' image in Diego Muñoz Camargo's *Descripción de la ciudad y provincia de Tlaxcala* [Description of the city and province of Tlaxcala] (c. 1581–84). The image, made by unacknowledged artists who worked alongside Muñoz Camargo, captured individual features and attributes of Aztec deities in the moment just prior to being ignited, having the paradoxical effect of safeguarding them from complete erasure.

9 According to Nemser: 'Even where the Spanish did not perceive American space as empty—the marvelous view of Tenochtitlan afforded to Cortés and Bernal Díaz del Castillo, for example, stands out—the urban materials accumulated there appeared to have a different character than their European counterparts. In colonial space, these residues of human life were not seen as deeply rooted but as strikingly superficial, easy to sweep away and replace or reorganize' (2017, 32).

text was truly rescued from oblivion by important Mexican intellectuals who recast Cárdenas as a solidary witness to the genesis of their regional identity. In an essay entitled 'Notas sobre la inteligencia americana' [Notes on the American intelligence] famed scholar Alfonso Reyes referred to him as a 'peninsular sage' whose work was an 'early literary testimony' of the 'new American way' [modo de ser americano] (1958, 304). Historian Emilio Uranga went a step further in his essay 'Juan de Cárdenas: his friends and enemies' counting himself among the former and calling the work 'the most Mexican book of the sixteenth century' (1991, 48). The author of the *Problemas y secretos* was a kindred spirit, Uranga declared to the audience attending the first Mexican conference on the History of Science held in 1964: 'Juan de Cárdenas is my mate' [mi cuate] (1964, 71). These affinities were motivated by the link that Reyes and Uranga saw between Cárdenas's defence of the intellectual prowess of the 'Spaniards of Mexico' and twentieth-century notions on Latin American and Mexican identity as they understood them (discussed in chapter 2). But while these readings were valuable in that they recognised the need to look past the seventeenth century into the region's older history, and to widen our selection of materials when tracing the origins of a Latin American mentality, if the goal is not merely to historicise how that nineteenth-century proposition was assumed over time but to retain it as a viable identitary category, then taking Cárdenas's position for an early paragon of that collective ethos is highly problematic since it requires that we actively disavow Indigenous, African and mixed race sites of enunciation for the Latin American experience.

Furthermore, reducing Cárdenas's identity to that of a peninsular observer also distorts the historical record somewhat, making him into an almost visitor, an impartial outsider who had the presence of mind to support the *criollo* cause, as it were, rather than seeing him as a full member of New Spain's diverse sixteenth-century community, which included many *radicados* like him. Reyes's reading effectively forces Cárdenas out of the place where he grew up and built his life, and where he did not feel a foreigner. As discussed earlier (see chapter 2), the author of the *Problemas y secretos* had arrived in the New World in his early teens and was educated locally, first with the Jesuits and then at the University of Mexico. Compared to the other authors of medical texts printed in Mexico in the sixteenth century, namely Bravo, Hinojosos and Farfán, not only did Cárdenas belong to a younger generation but, unlike them, he was a product of New World educational institutions through and through.[10] Likewise, as we would recall, for him there was but one *nación*: the Spanish, and Spaniards were either 'born in Spain' or 'born in the Indies', with the common link between them maintained despite a

10 As mentioned in chapter 3, although Farfán received a degree from the University of Mexico, it is unlikely he trained there. Pardo Tomás deduces Cárdenas studied at the Colegio Máximo de San Pedro y San Pablo given his mention of Antonio Rubio who taught there (2011b, 5).

difference in temperament (see chapter 2). The connection worked both ways, for if Spaniards born in the Indies shared a common constitution with those of Europe, writers born in Spain but who lived in the Americas, like him, were not to be prevented from partaking of a local identity. Although Cárdenas professed that he had less of a duty to write about the New World than those who had been born there, from an epistemological standpoint, he believed he had just as much authority to take on that task, an insider status he denied to Spaniards who remained in Spain and wrote about his home without having seen it first-hand.

Published when he was in his late 20s, the *Problemas y secretos* is a highly structured project and one that was not conceived first and foremost as a book on medicine, even though it was written by a physician. As Domingo Ledezma has observed, Cárdenas 'describes his work as one on natural history', situated within the humanist tradition, and 'manifest[ing] in it a purpose that goes beyond the practical and therapeutic elements of his profession' (2009, 153). It is organised into three parts: the first, a description of the land, the minerals and the winds; the second, a discussion on the flora and fauna of Mexico, including an extended description on the benefits of chocolate; and the third focuses on the people of New Spain. It conforms to the medieval genre of the *problemata*, which had become popular again in the sixteenth century, a connection disclosed in the title that, according to Luis Millones Figueroa, sought to 'unmarvel' or 'de-marvel' the secrets of the New World (2002, 90). *Problematas* typically entertained a selection of queries that would then lead to full explanations on causes and effects. The answers provided tended to incorporate possible caveats that were neutralised and explained away, thus giving the impression of a complete and fair discussion on the subject. The headings in Cárdenas's book articulate the *problemata*'s questions: 'Why does cocoa have a heating effect on the body despite being a cold substance?' (1591, fol. 105v); 'Why do trees in the Indies never lose their leaves, like those of Spain?' (1591, fol. 33v). Cárdenas's answers alternate between the impersonal and the first person ('about the first point I respond that ...' (1591, fol. 34r) or 'of what has been stated it is inferred that ...' (1591, fol. 149v)). However, seldom do these sections volunteer autobiographical statements that tie them to specific events in his life. In this he departs not only from Benavides, Hinojosos and Farfán, but also from Monardes and even Acosta, taking readers closer to encyclopaedic projects like those of Laguna and Covarrubias in their detached stance before their subject matter. Therefore, the moments where that conceit is either abandoned or minimised through the use of rhetorical structures are of particular interest since they allow us to better outline the coordinates of Cárdenas's discursive platform.

One such instance appears in the short prologue to the second book of the *Problemas y secretos* where Cárdenas expresses his gratitude to Juan de la Fuente, the University of Mexico's first professor of medicine. He calls Fuente 'a father', not just to him but to 'all of us who study in this [medical] faculty', a group he sets in opposition to 'the students in those universities in

Europe' with access to a panoply of resources unavailable in Mexico (1591, fol. 79v). He continues by explaining that, although 28 at the time of writing the prologue, he had composed the book when he was 26 years old, and that 'of those [years], half [he had] lived in Castile and half in the Indies' (1591, fol. 80r).[11] This information is shared in the context of the rhetorical *parvitas* whereby his readers were asked to forgive any shortcomings in the pages ahead on account of his youth and inexperience. But Cárdenas then abruptly adopts the position of an *epitimetikos*, which in classical rhetoric allowed for 'either a curse [to be] pronounced against a rival or thanks [to be] given to the audience' (Bruster and Weimann, 2004, 11). He uses this rhetorical window to lash out at potential critics who would question his right to speak:

> In my defence, it should also be considered how few authors I can turn to for support in what I write, since this is subject matter that has never been written about or shared by another, and the template that I have to articulate these responses is my own poor imagination, and with her I run the risk that many (because of my profession) will speak ill of me or behind my back; but in the end I take comfort in the fact that, good or bad, despite them being born and raised in the Indies and being older, more experienced and with greater means than I, they have not risen to the occasion, preferring to spend their efforts in the pomp and embellishment of their persons rather than in preaching and bringing to light the mysterious greatness of this fertile, grandiose and opulent land.[12]

The target of his remarks are not readers abroad ready to dismiss his findings on account of being those of a 'filósofo indiano' as he had described the role in the prologue, but rather intellectual figures belonging to his own geographic and social milieu, and more specifically, the *criollo* members of New Spain's society that he defends elsewhere.

At the same time that the *Problemas y secretos* acknowledges and discusses the period's debate about Spaniards born in the continent versus those born in the Indies, it is just as important to see how in his book Cárdenas argues strongly for a definition of identity that exceeds the accident of birth. The

11 José Pardo Tomás updates Cárdenas biography following Viesca Treviño and concludes he would have written the *Problemas y secretos* between his graduating in March 1589 and when he obtained his doctorate in 1590 (2011b, 5–6).

12 'También traigo por disculpa los pocos autores que tengo de quien sacar lo que escribo, porque como ésta es materia jamás escrita ni ventilada por otro, el dechado que tengo para dar estas respuestas es mi sola y pobre imaginación, y ella es la que me pone a riesgo de que muchos (y por ventura de mi oficio) tengan que murmurar y detraer de mí; pero al fin me consuelo que, malo o bueno, con ser ellos nacidos y criados en Indias y tener mucho más posible, edad y experiencia que yo, no han sido para otro tanto, estimando en más la pompa y ornamento de sus personas que el predicar y sacar a luz las misteriosas grandezas de esta fértil, grandiosa y opulenta tierra' (1591, fols. 80r–80v).

moorings of a colonial subject's identity and his entitlement to a discursive platform may have been anchored in a local experience but they were shaped and defined by their sense of allegiance to a community. *Peninsulares* were not all the same. It was not only *gachupines* who were scorned and mocked by locals—a group that could include *criollos*, *radicados* or seasoned visitors (see, for example, Benavides's treatment of *gachupines* in chapter 1)—, portraying them as newcomers dismissive of what they believed were impressive, hard-earned civilisational gains in a formerly 'barbarous' setting; they also resented administrators representing the Crown's interests: either short- or long-time residents of New Spain who because of their social and political status adopted a socially detached stance that exacerbated local anxieties about *calidad* and power in colonial hierarchies. As Arndt Brendecke explains referring to this group:

> [t]he viceroys, oidores, corregidors, and alcaldes mayores, and even the children of these officials, were forbidden from marrying persons coming from the particular administrative district where they served. ... Philip II expressly ordered that oidores and their wives were not to cultivate any friendships. They were also not allowed to take part in weddings or burials or even act as godfather. [These measures] were not aiming so much at maximal objectivity as they were at keeping the loyalty of the official as weak as possible toward his social environment. (2–16, 722–23)

Cárdenas, however, like the other writers of medical texts in New Spain, belonged to a category of *peninsulares* who were neither *gachupines* nor members of this more insulated social echelon. His expressions of friendship and gratitude towards his teachers, and the resentment that sometimes comes across when he refers to detractors, which the text always partly associates with *criollo* voices, belie a more complex image of the *peninsular* figure in New Spain at this juncture.

Whereas the tension between *peninsulares* and *criollos* still colours how we understand the region's history, and without minimising the importance of this opposition in shaping local structures and attitudes in the centuries that followed, the sixteenth-century portraits of colonial subjects that emerge in the *Problemas y secretos* call attention to the complex role of the *radicados*, figures whose profiles changed throughout the colonial era with succeeding waves of immigrants relocating to the Americas under different conditions. They are especially relevant to our discussion given their overrepresentation as authors of local imprints, including of all the medical texts printed in Mexico in the sixteenth century. But part of what makes them a useful focal point for a discussion on identity and self-fashioning is that their views are difficult to pin down in the *peninsular/criollo* divide, reflecting instead positions that were still being defined. In Cárdenas's case, for instance, his text did not go into multiple editions nor is there evidence that he wrote other books, despite mentioning in the *Problemas y secretos* that a second part of that work focused on Peru was forthcoming and notwithstanding that he continued to be active in New

Spain well into his 40s.[13] Elements of his biography hint at the possibility that his experience as a *radicado* coming of age in Mexico was considerably different from that of Hinojosos or Farfán. Cárdenas aspired to teach medicine at university level and writing the *Problemas y secretos* was surely an achievement he hoped would bring him closer to that goal. José Pardo Tomás is right to suggest that the praise he lavishes on *criollos* in some sections of his text are signs that he 'hoped to find patrons, patients, and a clientele that would enable him to live from medical practice' with the book aimed as 'a vehicle to attain prestige and legitimacy … in that specific context of the colonists' (2011b, 9). However, evidence is mixed on whether this is what happened, and whether his book was received in the way he perhaps intended. Cárdenas applied three times to the post of professor of medicine, first to the *cátedra de prima* when Fuente died in 1595, and then to the *cátedra de vísperas* when it was added to the curriculum in 1598; he was passed over in favour of other candidates both times. It would only be after Juan de Plasencia's death in 1607 that he would finally succeed in obtaining the *cátedra de vísperas* which he occupied for just two years until his death in 1609.[14] Whereas there is evidence that the *Problemas y secretos* was read after Cárdenas's death and there is an argument to be made for how, along with authors like Cervantes de Salazar and Bernardo de Balbuena, Cárdenas's writing demonstrates how seventeenth-century colonial rhetoric appropriated and refashioned many of the tropes and strategies first rehearsed by *radicados* in order to articulate *criollo* sensibilities, it would be other authors that readers would turn to in the last decade of the sixteenth century and first years of the next.[15]

One important text that set Cárdenas's ideas to a new agenda was Baltasar Dorantes de Carranza's *Sumaria relación de las cosas de la Nueva España con noticia individual de los descendientes legítimos de los conquistadores y primeros pobladores españoles* [Summary account of the things of New Spain with individual information on the legitimate descendants of the conquerors and

13 García Icazbalceta notes that some scholars believed there existed another text by Cárdenas on the topic of chocolate (see García Icazbalceta, 1954, 401 and Ledezma, 2009, 51). Somolinos d'Ardois believes this work never existed and may be an allusion to Book 2 of the *Problemas y secretos* which deals with that subject (Somolinos d'Ardois, 1980a, 298). Pardo Tomás agrees with Viesca Treviño's view that Cárdenas may have gone to Guadalajara, then capital of New Galicia, between 1599 and 1607 (2011b, 7).

14 The information on Cárdenas's teaching career is drawn from the archival work of Germán Somolinos d'Ardois rather than my direct consultation of archives. See Somolinos d'Ardois, 1980a, 207–08.

15 I refer here to the two printings of Farfán's text in 1592 and 1610 respectively, to the 1595 edition of Hinojosos's work, and also to a text that exceeds the parameters of the present study but that would be relevant in this context as well, the work of another *radicado*, Juan de Barrios's *Verdadera medicina, cirvgia, y astrologia en tres libros dividida* [The true medicine, surgery and astrology divided into three books], printed in Mexico City in 1607.

first Spanish settlers] (1604), a work that Stephanie Merrim describes as 'the prime inaugural manifestation of the creole-constructed Mexican archive' (2010, 135). Dorantes's reading of the *Problemas y secretos* homed in on the elements that best supported his main purpose, which was to '[carve] out a genealogy and a "position of space and authority within colonial society" for creoles' (Merrim, citing Higgins, 2010, 135). Dorantes was, after all, the son of Andrés Dorantes, the one-time companion of explorer Álvar Núñez Cabeza de Vaca and part of a generation that had seen their fortunes and social standing increasingly eroded due to the intrusion of colonial and ecclesiastical authorities, particularly in matters that pertained to the rights and obligations of Indigenous communities toward them. The phrasing of his title, with its adversarial stance in support of the 'legitimate' descendants of the conquistadors, positioned the text against the a priori backdrop of a challenge to that legitimacy. Dorantes spoke with a voice not unlike that of Díaz del Castillo from his father's generation who had insisted his retelling of the conquest of Mexico was true in a way that royal chronicler Francisco López de Gómara's was not, seeking to raise his account above others that enjoyed official support but lacked direct contact with the reality of the Americas.[16] The *Sumaria* drew on the *Problemas y secretos*'s defence of New World natural products and of *criollos* along a path that eventually leads to appraisals like those by Reyes and Uranga.

But Dorantes's approach was not the only possible reading of Cárdenas going forward into the seventeenth century. While true that the text exceeded the aims of a medical treatise, it still discussed a wealth of information relevant to the practice of medicine and New World pharmacopoeia, and it was this scientific angle that interested Francisco Ximénez. A Dominican lay friar and nurse, Ximénez had been born in Aragon and had lived in Italy, Spain and Florida before finally settling in New Spain in 1605.[17] There he came across the work of Francisco Hernández, former 'Protomédico General de las Nuevas Indias' and the supervising figure in Hinojosos's dissections (see chapter 2). Hernández had been given the title of *protomédico* in 1570 and the Spanish Crown had placed him in charge of a botanical expedition to New Spain with the aim of compiling a full survey of natural products useful in medicine (Pardo Tomás, 2002, 144–45). The fruits of his extensive research were sent to Philip II's court: '10 folio volumes of coloured paintings and six of verbal descriptions of 3000 plants, 40 quadrupeds, 229 birds, 58 reptiles, 30 insects, 54 aquatic animals [as well as] 35 minerals, and also

16 Díaz del Castillo described his work as the 'true' version of events (*Historia verdadera de la conquista de la Nueva España* (1551–84) [True history of the conquest of New Spain]) and denounced López de Gómara's *Historia General de las Indias*, first printed in 1552 and subsequently expanded, as false and incomplete. For a fuller discussion of Dorantes's reading of Cárdenas, see Merrim, 2010, 135–46.

17 Information on Ximénez's biography comes from the introduction written by Nicolás León in his 1888 edition of Hernández's text. See in particular pages vi–xi.

dried Aztec plants' (Egerton, 2004, 113). But the publication that would have disseminated Hernández's findings ran into a series of problems, including a shift in Spain's policies toward overseas territories in 1577, which banned printing literature on Indigenous groups and their customs (Brendecke, 2016, 537). As Brendecke explains, after Hernández's return to Spain, it was Antonio Sánchez de Renedo, the *protomédico* of Peru, who would be entrusted with continuing Hernández's efforts in the New World, and back in Spain, others were given a more salient role in bringing the editorial project to fruition (2016, 537).[18] Antonio Nardo Recchi, then a royal physician, was placed in charge of editing Hernández's work to prepare it for publication, but Hernández's and Recchi's deaths halted that effort. Hernández's research would instead be disseminated throughout Europe in a fragmentary way, including through a partial edition published in Rome in 1628 as the *Rerum medicarum Novae Hispaniae thesaurus*, as well as through notes taken by scholars from Hernández's originals which remained housed in El Escorial, and which were eventually destroyed in the fire of 1671. Recchi's version would be 'extremely important, because it was the basis for most of the dissemination of Hernández for two centuries' (Chabrán and Varey, 2000, 5), and it was a manuscript copy of this work that made its way back to the New World and into the hands of Ximénez who translated it from Latin into Spanish.[19] The *Quatro libros de la naturaleza, y virtudes de las plantas, y animales que estan receuidos en el vso de Medicina en la Nueva España, y la Methodo, y correccion y preparacion, quepara administrallas se requiere con lo que el Doctor Francisco Hernandez escriuio en lengua Latina* [Four books on the nature and virtues of plants and animals useful in Medicine in New Spain, and on the Method, exactitude and preparation that is required to administer them following what Doctor Francisco Hernández wrote in the Latin language] would be published in Mexico in 1615.

Ximénez explained that his motivation for undertaking the translation of Hernández rested on two main reasons: first, that despite the great wealth in medicinal products of the land and their increasing circulation overseas, knowledge about how to properly put them to use and make them into

18 For recent appraisals on the subject of Hernández's work and the dissemination of materials related to his research in Europe, see Eamon, 2019, 100–02 and Marroquín Arredondo, 2019, 45–69.

19 Scholars are divided on an assessment of how much Recchi's intervention changed Hernández's text. For example, Pardo Tomás points out that Hernández had tried to organise the material following Nahuatl names, giving a sense of Indigenous taxonomies, whereas Recchi's version had reassembled the material using Dioscorides as its template (2002, 160). Chabrán and Varey dispute the claim that Recchi's version distorted Hernández's work, arguing that his intervention 'did not seriously mar the original text' and only placed it into what they see as a coherent structure (2000, 5). Ximénez's own statement claims that Recchi had summarised it [moderola en menos volumen] (1615, viii).

medicines was lacking; and, second, that the information published up to that point about them was incorrect because it failed to understand 'our language', by which he meant a *criollo* discourse purporting to have already successfully decoded and absorbed Indigenous knowledge and able to navigate with ease the catalogue of Indigenous names (mostly in Nahuatl) for American flora and fauna. A by now familiar figure is singled out as a prime example of the circulation of misinformation:

> first because so few have written on this, and second because of the difficulty entailed in understanding our language and land which brings about many inconveniences, a reason that explains the errors committed by Doctor Monardes who was the first one who wrote on the singularity of the Indies in this regard, since what he said followed the information as was told to him by others.[20]

With the most backhanded of praises Ximénez adds: 'I commend him for his solicitous ability and intellect, that my goal is not to criticise another's work, but to declare according to my own limited knowledge the prerogatives and excellent properties of the natural remedies of the land.'[21] The problem according to Ximénez was that Monardes had simply got too much wrong and 'there was much to correct'.[22] In his introduction he also mentioned 'el Doctor fr. Augustín Farfán' as well as 'Alonso López de Hinojosos, de la Compañía, y muchos otros', but did so in an accusatory manner, implying their use of Hernández's ideas in their texts had been detrimental, leading to further confusion about proper procedures and medicines.[23] Cárdenas

20 'lo uno por ser pocos los que en esta materia han escrito, lo otro por la dificultad que trae consigo el conocimiento de cosas ajenas a nuestro lenguaje y tierra, cosa que trae consigo muchos inconvenientes, razón que disculpa los yerros que cometió el doctor Monardes, que fue el primero que las singularidades de las Indias en esta manera escribió, que lo que dijo fue según le refirieron los que las llevaban' (1615, viii).

21 'alabo su solícita habilidad, e ingenio que mi fin no es reprender escritos, sino declarar según mi poco caudal, las prerrogativas y excelencias de los remedios naturales de la tierra' (1615, viii).

22 'había mucho que enmendar' (1615, viii).

23 Skaarup's (2015, 223) is correct to suggest that Ximénez is denouncing that Hernández has been amply plagiarised ('pedazos de ha[n] aprovechado[e] impreso muchos doctores' ['parts have been appropriated and printed by many doctors'], 1615, xiii) but I disagree that he is extending that accusation to Farfán and Hinojosos. His point then seems to be more about how he believes they have corrupted Hernández's ideas rather than an accusation of the author having gone unacknowledged. Ximénez would have been aware that both Farfán and Hinojosos mentioned Hernández in their texts, it being particularly important for Hinojosos to have done so (as discussed in chapter 2). Ximénez's own collaborative role as translator and restorer of Hernández's ideas, and his own plagiarising of Cárdenas (to be discussed in the pages that follow) suggest a different set of objections in this regard.

he acknowledged by name once in folio 67v, yet, as I will show, Ximénez's translation of Hernández will borrow heavily from sources like the *Problemas y secretos* without signalling to the reader that he was adding material not his own.

In the *Quatro libros*'s section on the chewing of tzictli[24] Ximénez clarifies that this practice did not have the same stimulating effects as chewing coca or tobacco leaves; quite the opposite, he argues, the face and even the whole body could become tired from the repetitiveness of the activity. The text then digresses into a passage on the relationship between digestion and alertness that is presented almost as if it were gossip, something too compelling not to share:

> But, well, it is so relevant, that although I digress, I want to go on a little bit more, and thus I say that regardless of how long one chews food in the mouth, if it does not go to the stomach to be digested and cooked and distributed after to all the body, it cannot provide nourishment, and all this seems to contradict the verdict and opinion of a very modern newly invented book. It says there that as the food is chewed in the mouth it nourishes the body through the smoke that rises from the food to the brain and is distributed to all the body and it nourishes the body as is known, it says there, by experience.[25]

This 'little bit more' turns out to be a critique of a 'new' unspecified text. According to his summary, this source claimed that food did not have to pass through the stomach to provide nourishment and that instead the 'smoke' released in the act of chewing was enough. Ximénez does not reveal the author that purportedly made such a claim; for that information, we would have to go to the section of Cárdenas's *Problemas y secretos* that he turns out to be plagiarising:

> But, well, it is so relevant, that although I digress, I want to go on a little bit more; I said at the top of this chapter that the food, regardless of how long it is chewed in the mouth, if it does not go to the stomach and from there to be digested and cooked and distributed throughout the body once cooked, it cannot provide nourishment.[26]

24 The etymological source for the Spanish 'chicle' [chewing gum].

25 'Pero pues viene tan a cuento, quiero aunque sea algo prolijo alargarme un poquito más, y así digo que el manjar por más que se masque en la boca, como no vaya al estómago, y allí se digera y se cueza y se reparta despues de cocido a todo el cuerpo, no puede dar sustento, todo esto parece que contradice a la sentencia, y parecer de un libro muy moderno nuvuamente inuentado dice allí, que mientras el manjar se masca en la boca da sustento al cuerpo, por cuanto aquellos humos que suben del manjar al cerebro se reparten a todo el cuerpo y estos le dan luego sustento como se conoce según allí dice. Por la experiencia' (1615, fol. 97v).

26 'Pero pues viene tan a cuento, quiero, aunque sea algo prolijo, alargarme un poquito más; yo dije en el remate de este capítulo que el manjar, por más que se mascase

The acknowledgment of sources in early colonial New World historiography is a complex issue, for even though personal experience played an increasingly important role in authorising knowledge epistemologically, demonstrating familiarity with texts that were relevant at the time in Europe, both ancient, like Dioscorides, and contemporary, like Monardes, was a way of linking locally produced information to a wider conversation. As Kevin Perromat Augustín has argued, there is an 'apparent contradiction [in] the study of American historiography' for on the one hand, there is an acknowledgment of what constitutes plagiarism and a 'persistent enunciation of citation conventions at work during the period' that goes hand in hand with a 'simultaneous and persistent ignoring of [these conventions]' (2010, 153). In Ximénez's case, his decision to not disclose that he is quoting Cárdenas is ironic given his complaints about how Hernández's work had been appropriated.

If we compare the two passages cited above, we see that Ximénez reproduces Cárdenas's sentence structure, vocabulary and cadence almost verbatim, following him even in the choice of using diminutives to preserve the mocking tone with which these novel ideas are treated. Yet the omissions he makes are telling, as we see when the original passage is read in full:

> and all this seems to contradict the verdict of doña Oliva Sabuco, which is a newly invented book. It says there that as the food is chewed in the mouth it nourishes the body, because the smoke that rises from the food to the brain is distributed throughout the body and thus feeds it as is known, according to her, by experience, for we see that if a man is tired and as they say, dying of hunger, just by beginning to chew the sustenance, before it is cooked in the stomach, already his limbs begin to gain strength.[27]

Neither Sabuco's identity, nor the detail that the source is a female author, is conveyed in Ximénez's unacknowledged paraphrase, which continues all the way to Cárdenas's hypothetical test of her scientific conclusions. In the *Problemas y secretos*, it reads:

> Indeed, that if this opinion, or fantasy, were true, that the human body can survive from smoke, I would dare suggest feeding an entire monastery of friars only with the scent of a hearty stew, leaving it as full as it was before, since without eating, by bringing their mouths and noses closer to

en la boca, como no fuese al estómago y de allí se digiriese y cociese repartiéndose después de cocido a todo el cuerpo, no podía dar sustento' (1591, fols. 136v–137r).

27 'todo esto parece que contradice a la sentencia de doña Oliva Sabuco, que es un libro nuevamente inventado, dice allí que mientras que el manjar se masca en la boca da sustento al cuerpo, por cuanto aquellos humos que suben del manjar al cerebro se reparten por todo el cuerpo y éstos le dan luego sustento, como se conoce, según ella dice, por la experiencia, pues vemos que si un hombre está desmayado y muerto, como dicen, de hambre, en comenzando a mascar el mantenimiento, antes de ser cocido en el estómago, se comienzan a reforzar y alegrar los miembros del cuerpo' (1591, fol. 137r).

its vapours, a hefty quantity of such vapours or smoke could reach the brain from which they could sustain themselves, although I fear that they will be left just as hungry as before.[28]

It is easy to see why this section caught Ximénez's eye in the first place, as the images of the 'good stew' and of a monastery chockfull of famished friars highlight the passage especially in the context of the *Problemas y secretos* as a whole, since for the most part, and unlike Benavides or Farfán, Cárdenas's prose is seldom sarcastic or funny. At first glance it would seem his dismissal of Sabuco is an unsurprising instance of patriarchal attitudes of the period undermining women's intellectual capabilities. Indeed, the section comes to an end with the author's refusal to engage in any further consideration of the text: 'and thus I offer', writes Cárdenas, 'that this opinion of doña Oliva is as true as the rest of the inventions her book contains',[29] discarding by association any other possible contribution she stood to offer. But while there is a case to be made for him using her first name rather than her last name to address her ('doña Oliva') as a derisive gesture, and that this in and of itself constitutes a dismissive treatment based on her sex, arguably what is more surprising is that this is as far as it goes if so. Cárdenas launches no explicit attacks on Sabuco on the basis of her gender. No expression of surprise is shared with readers at the fact a recently published book bearing what would be a living female author's name, and on the subject of human health, was circulating in Spain and in Mexico City. Neither did Cárdenas question Sabuco's authorship in the *Problemas y secretos*, but rather took issue with what seemed to him her hopelessly flawed epistemological methods.

The author of the *Nveva filosofia dela natvraleza del hombre, no conocida, ni alcançada de los grandes filosofos antiguos: la qual mejora la vida y salud humana* (1587) [New philosophy of human nature: neither known nor attained by the ancient philosophers, which will improve human life and health], was born in Alcaraz in 1562, the daughter of Miguel Sabuco, a pharmacist and local public servant (see figure 4.1b). Twenty-five years old and already married when the *Nveva filosofia* first appeared, the text would be republished the following year with some sections censored by the Inquisition, and was issued twice more before the end of the sixteenth century. In it was offered an evaluation of medical practice from the vantage point of personal experience,

28 'Por cierto que si esta opinión o imaginación fuera verdad de que el cuerpo humano se sustentara de humo, que me atreviera yo a sustentar con sólo el olor de una buena olla a todo un convento de frailes, quedándose la olla tan entera como estaba de antes, porque sin comer de ella podían, llegando la boca y narices a aquel vapor, subir gran suma de tal vapor o humo al cerebro y sustentarse con él, pero entiendo quedaran tan muertos de hambre como de antes' (1591, fols. 137r–137v). Cárdenas enhances the humour of the passage with the semantic wordplay on the phrase 'muerto de hambre', which also means to be a beggar, or a 'nobody'.

29 'así que yo esta opinión de doña Oliva juzgo por tan verdadera como otras invenciones que en su libro trae' (1591, fol. 137v).

which was then presented as a guide for maintaining good health by avoiding activities that brought on premature death, namely illness and poor habits. It was structured as a series of seven colloquies between the shepherds Antonio, Rodonio and Veronio, who discussed medical matters in a *locus amoenus*, joined by a fourth character, a physician, who enters in treatise 5. Like Huarte de San Juan, Sabuco divided human nature into three parts: the vegetative soul which is shared with the plant world, the sentient soul, which is shared with animals, and the rational soul, which is shared with angels and divine beings. Premature death and health problems were caused by a series of affects (anger, sorrow, rage, sadness, love, desire and fear) that the individual was able to control by means of self-knowledge. The brain played a key role in maintaining the health of the body as arbiter of its physiological processes.

Sabuco's text was reprinted every century thereafter, with at least a dozen known editions, but the work is not without controversy.[30] Early in the twentieth century, Miguel Sabuco's will came to light and in it he claimed that he, and not his daughter, had been the author of the *Nveva filosofia*. Unfortunately, the critical work done around that time to see how the discovery of this archival document fit into a historical context does not resolve the issue by present-day standards and partook of notions about gender and intellectual ability that no longer hold. Scholars like Mary Ellen Waithe and Dámaris Otero-Torres have argued strongly that the document needs to be studied in relation to an ongoing family dispute between father, daughter and Oliva's brother.[31] They point out also that her authorship does not seem to have been questioned by her contemporaries but rather the opposite, with figures of high standing at the time like Lope de Vega referring to Sabuco as a 'tenth muse'. In her letter of dedication to Philip II, Sabuco referred to herself as a 'humble female serf and vassal' who 'dares to speak' to 'ask for protection and shelter under the aquiline wings of Your Majesty, under which take this, my son which I have begotten' (Sabuco, 2007, 44).[32]

30 Present-day scholarship on Sabuco is sharply divided, and the problem has been further compounded as a result of recent competing editorial projects and translations produced independently of one another. The most thorough and thoughtful consideration of the matter to date remains Beatriz Cruz-Sotomayor's PhD dissertation, *'Tan estraño y nuevo es el libro, quanto es el autor': autoría y recepción en la Nueva filosofia de Oliva Sabuco* (2008) which weighs the evidence fairly, and examines also what would be the implications of a male figure taking on a female writing persona in the literary and social context of late sixteenth-century Madrid.

31 See the introduction in Waithe, Vintró and Zorita's edition of the *New Philosophy* (2007).

32 The original passage reads: 'Una humilde sierva y vasalla, hincadas las rodillas en ausencia, pues no puede en presencia, osa hablar … [para] pedir el amparo y sombra de las Aquilinas alas de V. C. M. debajo de las cuales pongo este mi hijo que yo he engendrado … Y aunque la cesárea y católica majestad tenga dedicados muchos libros de hombres, a lo menos de mujeres pocos y raros, y ninguno de esta materia. Tan extraño y nuevo es el libro, cuanto es el autor' (1587, fols. 1r–2r).

The selection of Philip II as addressee was not surprising if one considers the monarch's reputation at the time as a patron of the sciences. Eamon, who characterises the period's Spanish court as 'a magnet for natural philosophers' notes that '[c]ontrary to the opinion that seems to prevail among non-Spanish historians of science, the royal court in Madrid was alive with scientific activity. Philip was deeply interested in the sciences of the day and spent lavishly on scientific pursuits' (2005, 4, 11). From his support of the Casa de la Contratación, to his funding of Hernández's scientific expedition, to his hosting of scientific minds on the forefront of innovation, such as Vesalius and Leonardo Fioravanti, Sabuco's text surfaced at a time and place where it would not have been seen as a peripheral effort for pertaining to medicine and science.[33] The issue of female authorship is addressed directly in the dedication and linked to the notion of innovation: 'even if your Caesarean and Catholic Majesty has had many books dedicated to Him from men, only few and rare have been by women, and none about this subject matter' (Sabuco, 2007, 44). Even so, there are signs that Sabuco's authorship was questioned as far back as the eighteenth century, and there are unanswered questions about how material that has been taken as conclusive proof of a female writer fits within the *Querelle des femmes*.[34] The mention of the *Nveva filosofia* in the *Problemas y secretos* adds a new, American page to this ongoing debate underscoring the quick circulation of Iberian print materials relating to medicine in early colonial Mexico and, importantly, it also speaks to the place a book written by a woman could have had in the formative years of colonial intellectual life. Cárdenas's reading squarely places Sabuco among the very first women authors ever to be discussed in print in the Americas, even if he turns to her work in an attempt to discredit the accuracy of her conclusions.[35]

As in the texts by Benavides, Hinojosos, Farfán and Cárdenas, the *Nveva filosofia* also rested on the sixteenth-century epistemological framework that privileged direct experience, a point made in the text by the shepherd Antonio

33 Vesalius served Philip II's from 1559 to 1564 and had been a physician to his father, Charles V, to whom he had dedicated the *Fabrica*. Fioravanti was invited by Philip II to his court in 1576 and he later dedicated *Della fisica* (1582) to him.

34 For a critique of Waithe, Vintró and Zorita and a discussion that argues her authorship cannot be conclusively established, see the introduction in Pomata's edition of *The True Medicine* (2010).

35 The influence of Sabuco's work in New World writing is a matter that has not yet been addressed by scholars. Aside from a long footnote in Ángeles Durán's 1988 edition of the *Problemas y secretos*, the subject of the New World readers of the text remains unexplored. This would seem a necessary step in light of the fact that the *Nveva filosofia* appears in booksellers' stock lists alongside texts by other medical authors like Juan Fragoso (González Sánchez, 2011, 177). Ximénez's erasure of her name thus could be a clue to other instances where the Sabuco's ideas may have been discussed, even if her name was suppressed.

who, like Monardes (as discussed in chapter 1), also compared scientific enquiry with the Columbian enterprise:

> the beginning of a new thing is doubtful and difficult to admit in the minds of men, as was the case with Columbus's opinion at the time of the Catholic King Don Fernando, when he claimed that there was another world beyond the sea, which seemed to everybody so new and unheard-of that for a long time they did not believe him, until after much pressing they decided to try and find out through experience whether perchance the man was right. And thus his view was proved true and found to be right, as everybody knows. I ask the same trial and experience for my novelty. I don't want people to believe me but to believe the experience and truth of the thing itself. (2010, 98–99)[36]

Experience, confirmation, investigation, test, proof, truth; this vocabulary is ever-present in Sabuco and Cárdenas, and is at the heart of both authors' central claims. However, Sabuco pushes that position to the limit, arguing that anyone of sound judgment is qualified to generate knowledge, even about medical matters: 'Not only wise and Christian physicians may be the judges of it', offers Sabuco, 'but also anyone else of fair judgment versed in other disciplines and any capable person of good judgment' (2007, 45).[37] While the end of life was unavoidable, the *Nveva filosofia* maintained unnatural, premature death caused by illness was excessive; canonical medicine had failed humanity because it had neglected to show people how to properly care for their well-being. The justification for her project was to provide readers with information that would enable them to take control over their bodies. As she argues in the opening letter:

> For my petition is fair: to test my doctrine for one year. … Hippocrates' and Galen's medicine has been tested for two thousand years, and their results have been so ineffective and inconclusive, as we clearly see every day and as was seen during the great flu, spotted fever, smallpox, and

36 'No ignoro que todo principio de cosa nueva es dudoso, y dificultoso de ser admitido en la opinión de los hombres, como fue la que trajo Colón en tiempo del Emperador Carlos V cuando echó por la boca que había otro mundo de aquel cabo del mar. Lo cual les pareció a todos una cosa tan nueva y tan no hablada en el mundo que por mucho tiempo no le dieron crédito, hasta que por gran importunación quisieron probar y experimentar si acaso aquel hombre tenía razón en lo que decía, y así se probó, y se halló su verdad tan buena, como todos saben. La cual prueba y experiencia yo también pido en mi novedad, y no quiero que me crean a mí sino a la experiencia y verdad de la cosa' (1587, fols. 204v–205r). Pomata's translation clarifies that Sabuco's error of referring to Charles V rather than Ferdinand as king of Spain during Columbus's time was corrected in subsequent editions.

37 'no solamente los sabios y cristianos médicos pueden ser jueces, pero aun también los de alto juicio de otras facultades, y cualquier hombre hábil, y de buen juicio' (1587, fol. 3r).

> during many other illnesses where [medicine] does not work at all. Out of a thousand only three survive until natural death arrives. The others die violent deaths from illness, not having benefited from the old medicine. (2007, 45)[38]

Her call was for a more exact and comprehensive approach to maintaining good health, which is to be arrived at by means of personal experience.

Cárdenas's mention of the *Nveva filosofia* in the *Problemas y secretos* appears in the second part, in a chapter where he elucidates how and why chewing wards off hunger. He explains that while coca and tobacco were strong herbs and caused the person to feel intoxicated ('causan un género de embriaguez'), chewing other substances, like tzictli, which lacked those properties, was still able to draw phlegm to the mouth from the brain, which then made its way to the stomach and sustained the person, albeit without providing additional nourishment, which he claims is what Sabuco contends (1988, 166). That the discussion is centred not just on physiological processes but on New World substances is significant, as Cárdenas was contesting Sabuco's first-hand knowledge of them as someone writing in Spain rather than Mexico.[39] If we turn to the *Nveva filosofia*, Sabuco's model is less simplistic than the *Problemas y secretos* would make it appear, claiming not that the brain feeds on vapours alone, but that the process of digestion is two-fold and begins before the food arrives inside the stomach (Sabuco, 2007 [1587], 193). Cárdenas distorts her description, neglecting to mention Sabuco's obvious understanding of the important role played by that organ.

But if the information in the *Nveva filosofia* was so clearly flawed according to Cárdenas, why include it at all? Two reasons may have fuelled his critique. The first could be Sabuco's choice of a literary conceit in writing about physiology, with the character of a doctor being persuaded by the words of uneducated shepherds. Cárdenas, who so admired the dedication of Fuente to his profession, and given his nascent sense of pride in the quality of his education, would have been understandably irked both by a boastful character who dismissed the importance of institutionalised medical training and, especially, by what must have seemed as an unfair caricature of a member of his profession portrayed as being in awe of the shepherds'

38 'pues mi petición es justa, que se pruebe esta mi secta un año, pues han probado la medicina de Hipócrates y Galeno dos mil años, y en ella han hallado tan poco efecto y fines tan inciertos, como se ve claro cada día, y se vio en el gran catarro, tabardete, viruelas, y en pestes pasadas, y otras muchas enfermedades, donde no tiene efecto alguno, pues de mil no viven tres, todo el curso de la vida hasta la muerte natural: y todos los demás mueren muerte violenta de enfermedad, sin aprovechar nada su medicina antigua' (1587, fol. 4r).

39 The coca leaf had become a familiar product in the Hispanic world and appears in the works of Pedro Mártir de Anglería, Francisco López de Gómara and Pedro Cieza de León, among others. Cieza de León wrote that, as early as 1553, some merchants in Spain had become rich with the sale of the coca acquired from Indigenous markets.

logic. But secondly, and perhaps more to the point for him than a difference of opinion on the physiology of digestion, was Sabuco's problematic understanding of the notion of experience, and her use of the term, given that Cárdenas was also heavily invested in redefining what it meant from an epistemological standpoint. What counts as experience, and whose experience counts? This conundrum will become a chief preoccupation for New World scholars over the next two centuries, who felt increasingly excluded from a global intellectual community. Already in the work of a writer like Cárdenas are the seeds of a larger complaint about the peripheral role American modes of scientific thought would play, and the displacement of knowledge produced in the Americas, even as local products either became assimilated, or continued to be a source of interest for Europe, all the way to the expeditions of José Celestino Mutis, Alejandro Malaspina and Alexander von Humboldt. Cárdenas's informed treatment of European publications becomes typical of the opposite stance in Europe regarding overseas print culture. One of the reasons why Sabuco is treated so harshly in the *Problemas y secretos* may be linked to the fact that her characters professed to be followers of Monardes, the other source that will be strongly refuted by Cárdenas in his text and whose discursive platform on New World *materia medica* he will contest.

Monardes's *Historia medicinal* is clearly a source of several of the medical and botanical tenets Sabuco's book relies upon, but it goes one step further by having a fictional character refer directly to the Sevillian doctor in two of the conversations. 'Why then is it that the old medicine, being mistaken as you said, is then right for so many illnesses and cures them?', asks Veronio.[40] Is it possible to still rely on the certainties of old if their epistemological basis is being called into question? To which Antonio offers a detailed and reasoned answer supported by the *Historia medicinal*:

> Because, as I will explain, you should know that the human body heals through these channels and also heals with medicines that work through those channels or immediately expels the vicious brain humour upward through the skull and commissures of the scalp. … Because drinking the juice of this china root (exempli gratia) as Monardes says, cures and heals all kinds of *bubas*, old sores, ulcers, head contusions, birth defects, joint pains, gout, sciatica pain, persistent headaches, and stomach aches. It heals rheums, obstructions, oedema and facial pallor, jaundice, paralysis and nervous diseases.[41]

40 This passage is not included in the existing English translations of Sabuco, so I offer my own. The original reads: 'Pues cómo la medicina antigua estando tan errada como vos decís acierta en muchas enfermedades, y las sana?' (1587, fol. 187r).

41 'Porque habéis de saber que el cuerpo humano sana por estas vías que os diré, y medicinas que por ellas obran, o bota por arriba el humor vicioso de esta raíz por cráneo y comisuras al cuero … Porque si esta raíz de la china (exempli gratia) como

Antonio's reading of Monardes is thorough and accurate when compared against the original. The character will mention him again when explaining to his companion the process by which bezoars are effective, mirroring his hyperbolic and lyrical descriptions of the stones, the very same sections of the *Historia medicinal* that come under fire in the *Problemas y secretos*.

Of Monardes's ideas on bezoars, Cárdenas writes:

> Given that the very fine and precious bezoars had their first origin in the Indies it is fair that in a history of the Indies they ought to be mentioned, although not with all the praise that was lavished upon them by doctor Monardes, who was the first who so extolled and praised them, leaving us more to edit out than things to say about them, and thus setting aside all their virtues, if indeed they are as numerous as he says, I only want to declare the manner and order in which nature creates them inside of animals.[42]

For Monardes, bezoars were formed in certain animals that, when bitten by poisonous snakes, instinctually sought out medicinal herbs they knew to be antidotes. Then, if they went into a river and the temperature was just right, he claimed, the heat generated by the venom would be neutralised by the coldness of the water, forming the stone, which became lodged either in the stomach or in the tear ducts. Cárdenas denounces this view as rubbish, pointing out mockingly that animals are well kept in the Indies, and that their owners cannot afford to have them run around wild to drink at their leisure in springs, never to return. For him, bezoars are sediment formations arising from layers of material accumulated in the stomachs of some animals, and he is not persuaded that those of the New World are very useful in medicine. The language he uses to debunk Monardes's claim is the strongest in all of the negative assertions in the *Problemas y secretos*:

> Notice now how are we to believe an author who holds such an opinion [on how bezoars are formed] or foolishness that he would sell us as truth. Seeing how widespread this error is among common folk, I thought it wise to banish it from their minds with sufficient examples and reasons, establishing thus the truth and what actually takes place, and this [I do]

dice Monardes cura y sana su agua bebida todo género de bubas, llagas viejas, úlceras, tolondones, o malas nacidas, dolores de junturas, gota, ciática, dolor de cabeza antiguo y de estómago, sana las reumas, opilaciones, hidropesía, quita el mal color del rostro, sana la ictericia, sana perlesía, y toda enfermedad de nervios' (1587, fol. 187v).

42 'Pues las finísimas y muy preciosas bezoares tuvieron su primer origen en las Indias, justo será en historia de Indias tratar alguna cosa de ellas, aunque no con tantos encarecimientos como el doctor Monardes, que fue el que en tanto grado las encumbró y ensalzó, que más nos dejó que quitar que decir de ellas, y así dejando sus muchas virtudes aparte (si son tantas como él dice), quiero sólo declarar el modo y orden que naturaleza guarda en forjar dentro del animal estas bezoares' (1591, fols. 150v–151r).

> only to please and satisfy the curiosity of many that I see investigate such secrets in the Indies.[43]

The attack continues over the course of several pages, with growing impatience and disdain: 'bezoars do not form in tear ducts, as some have dreamt, that this business is better suited for telling jokes than for the page'.[44] As he had done with Sabuco, Cárdenas will find fault with the reasoning behind Monardes's points, claiming his flawed judgment extends to other areas of his work, despite the fact that elsewhere in the text he will espouse views that were actually shared by both, such as their agreement on the positive medicinal properties of tobacco.

If we compare Cárdenas's discussion on this plant with that of Hinojosos, another source that also makes mention of Monardes, a clearer picture appears of what is at stake in terms of colonial rhetoric. Whereas Cárdenas, like Monardes, defended the value of tobacco and lauded its potential health benefits, Hinojosos stood diametrically opposed to that view. As seen in chapter 2, Hinojosos's opportunity to dissect the body of a smoker in Oaxaca had arisen because colonial authorities had wanted the general populace to see the detrimental effects of smoking on the body which, as we recall, the *Svmma* deemed as devastating on the inner organs as cocoliste, turning everything black and obliterating their anatomical contours. Although less direct, Hinojosos's evaluation of Monardes on tobacco turns out to be as scathing as the one Cárdenas offers on bezoars. Hinojosos writes:

> While discussing picietl Monardes says that when the chieftains wanted to make a decision, they would throw picietl leaves in the fire, and they would inhale the smoke, and they would lose their senses, and there the devil would communicate what he wanted, to fool them. This is how he fools these poor men, making them believe they improve, and not only do they not improve but [inhaling picietl] leaves them dumb, as we see that the vapours are enough to cause heart problems.[45]

43 'Notad ahora cómo se puede dar crédito acerca de las virtudes de la bezoar al autor que semejante opinión o desatino nos quiere persuadir y vender por verdad. Viendo pues cuán creído y recibido está en el vulgo semejante yerro, me pareció con muy bastantes experiencias y razones desterrarlo de los entendimientos, y estableciendo en todo ello la verdad y lo que real y verdaderamente pasa, y esto no más para gusto y curiosidad de muchos que veo en las Indias escudriñar semejantes secretos' (1591, fols. 151v–152r).

44 'La piedra bezoar se engendra no en los lagrimales de los ojos, como soñaron algunos, que esto más es negocio para reír que para escribir' (1591, fol. 155v).

45 'Monardes tratando del piciete dice, que cuando a los caciques se les ofrecía algún negocio, que echaban las hojas del piciete en la lumbre, y chupaban el humo, y quedaban sin sentido, y que allí les comunicaba el demonio lo que quería, para engañarlos. Así engaña a estos míseros, háceles creer que mejoran, y no sólo no mejoran, antes los deja necios, como vemos que los vapores del cuerpo son bastantes a dar mal de corazón' (1595, fol. 151r).

Hinojosos had already referred to Monardes in passing in the 1578 edition of the *Svmma*, making no special positive or negative remarks. However, the discussion on tobacco is new to the 1595 version. The passage engages in a curious form of slippage where Monardes is brought in as a source of information on Indigenous divination practices. But the observation on false religious beliefs from a Christian standpoint is linked to medicinal claims. Hinojosos continues: 'that the smoke is a very harmful thing is clearly seen in the evidence, for it is worse for the body than pestilence, and for all this the devil has tricks, making them believe they are restored from their illnesses, and he deceives them, because they go about always choking and yellow'.[46] On the surface, the blame seems to lie with the chieftains who, in their ignorance, are misled by superstition. But a reader who is aware that the *Historia medicinal* not only described picietl but strongly advocated smoking as a practice with health benefits is able to detect the slight: is it the devil who fools people into believing smoking is beneficial and can cure illness, or is it Monardes?

Tellingly, although Cárdenas sides with Monardes on this point, as Pardo Tomás has noticed, he makes no mention of there being a common ground between them and underscores instead the originality of his contribution to medical knowledge: 'Cárdenas once again insisted on the novelty of his treatise', writes Pardo Tomás, 'especially in relation to the question of smoking tobacco, a "medicament that only came into use recently among the Spaniards, and about which nobody has written". It is hard to believe Cárdenas did not know the work of Nicolás Monardes' (2011b, 15). Given the careful treatment afforded to the subject of the bezoars, it would be difficult indeed to suggest Cárdenas had somehow missed the section on tobacco, which suggests the exclusion is deliberate. Therefore, whereas the people of New Spain would seem to be divided on the issue of smoking, with the university-trained doctor claiming it was beneficial on one side, and the nurse practitioner backed by colonial authorities disagreeing with that view in the strongest terms on the other, they stood united in not wanting an outsider like Monardes to speak on their behalf. Both agreed that Monardes was a peddler of fantasies, the same sentiment echoed by Ximénez even if his treatment of the *Svmma* and the *Problemas y secretos* in the *Quatro libros* is itself dubious.

By the time of the *Problemas y secretos*'s publication in 1591, multiple versions of Monardes's *Historia medicinal* had been printed (see figure 4.2a). It had been translated into Latin by Charles L'Ecluse (1574), into Italian by Annibale Briganti (1580), into French by Jacques Gohory (1588) and into English by John Frampton (1581), recast in that version as the *Joyfull Newes*

46 'Que el humo sea cosa bien pestilencial, bien se ve por evidencia, pues para los cuerpos peor es que la pestilencia, y para todo esto tiene astucias el demonio, haciéndoles creer que mejoran de sus enfermedades, y los engaña, porque siempre se andan ahogando, y amarillos' (1595, fol. 151r).

out of the Newe Founde Worlde. From its first publication in 1565 to the end of the century (and excluding copies that circulated in manuscript), it would have 25 editions in six languages, with 14 additional ones undertaken in the seventeenth century (López Piñero and López-Terrada, 1997, 56). While Cárdenas may have wished for a *tabula rasa* in 1591 on which he and other 'filósofos indianos' could write the story of the New World, European voices like Monardes had taken a definitive lead. Working outside official channels for gathering information, and displaced by sources produced in Europe, Cárdenas's book did not resonate with the wider European public nor with institutions like the Council of the Indies, which, as Brendecke has noted, showed no interest in acquiring American imprints.[47]

Indigenous literacies could be undervalued and ignored locally, but arguably the platform the *Problemas y secretos* contested most directly was that of overseas contemporaries, whose superior resources and access to mechanisms with which to record and share their findings created a rhythm of knowledge dissemination the writers of the New World could not compete with. Indeed, one of the few surviving copies of the *Problemas y secretos* that reached the Old World at the time, now housed at the British Library, shows traces of a reader from the period who doubted Cárdenas's claims on several occasions, and chose to highlight sections where the author had conceded some of the weaknesses of character attributed to the Spaniards of Mexico. For all the positive effects the environment had on their humoral constitution, Cárdenas had acknowledged it also resulted in a 'lack perseverance in their affairs, and thus we can truly say that in this land men have an excess of ingenuity but lack constancy and perseverance'.[48] This lead Catalonian financier Miguel Camarena to conclude that 'the people of the Indies are naturally untrustworthy', a sentiment he wrote on the margins of his personal copy in an instance of what could be termed 'hostile marginalia' (see figure 4.2b).[49] It is under these circumstances, with

47 Brendecke observes that, as of 1606 'the Council owned only eighteen books, including one on clerical and secular law, an edition with commentary of the *Siete Partidas*, the legal codification of the laws of America by Diego de Encinas, a book about the Council of Trent, the official instruction for the Casa de la Contratación, the *Leyes de Indias*, and a dictionary on the language of Peru' (2016, 655).

48 'haciéndoles poco perseverantes en sus cosas, y así realmente podemos decir que en esta tierra sobra en los hombres la viveza y falta la constancia y perseverancia' (1591, fol. 181v).

49 'La gen[te] de indi[as] es inco[ns]tante natu[ral]mente' reads the handwriting on folio 181r of the copy housed at the British Library. Sadly, this imprint was trimmed at some point in its binding history, making other comments by this reader difficult to decipher. In folio 241r, Camarena questions Cárdenas's assertion that worms and other vermin do not spontaneously arise from poorly digested food in the stomach, which the author dismisses in the *Problemas y secretos* as folk tales. Camarena feels differently about spontaneous generation and writes that, 'if this were true', neither foodstuffs like basil, eggplants nor 'an infinity of other herbs' would engender the

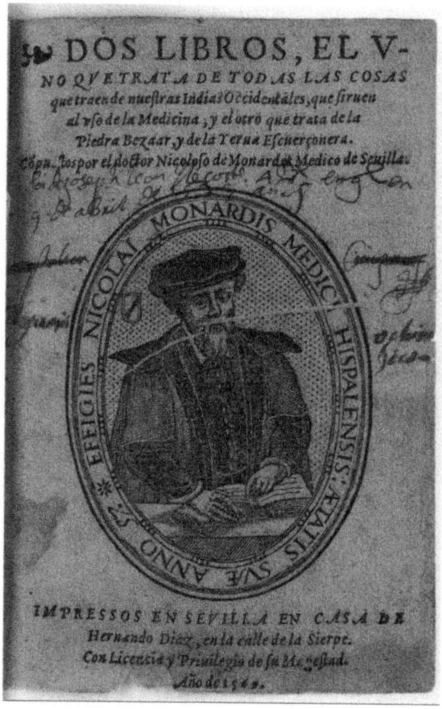

DOS LIBROS, EL V-
NO QVE TRATA DE TODAS LAS COSAS
que traen de nuestras Indias Occidentales, que siruen
al vso de la Medicina, y el otro que trata de la
Piedra Bezaar, y de la Yerua Escuerçonera.
Cōpu..tos por el doctor Nicoloso de Monardes Medico de Seuilla.

EFFIGIES NICOLAI MONARDIS MEDICI HISPALENSIS: AETATIS SVAE ANNO 52

IMPRESSOS EN SEVILLA EN CASA DE
Hernando Diaz, en la calle de la Sierpe.
Con Licencia y Priuilegio de su Magestad.
Año de 1569.

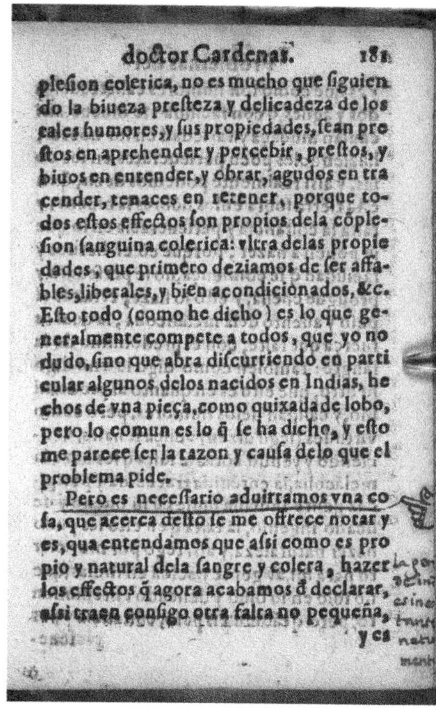

doctor Cardenas. 181

plesion colerica, no es mucho que siguien do la biueza presteza y delicadeza de los tales humores, y sus propiedades, sean prestos en aprehender y percebir, prestos, y biuos en entender, y obrar, agudos en tracender, tenaces en retener, porque todos estos effectos son propios dela cōplesion sanguina colerica: vltra delas propiedades, que primero deziamos de ser affables, liberales, y bien acondicionados, &c. Esto todo (como he dicho) es lo que generalmente compete a todos, que yo no dudo, sino que abra discurriendo en particular algunos delos nacidos en Indias, hechos de vna pieça, como quixada de lobo, pero lo comun es lo q̃ se ha dicho, y esto me parece ser la razon y causa delo que el problema pide.

Pero es necessario aduirtamos vna cosa, que acerca desto se me offrece notar y es, qua entendamos que assi como es propio y natural dela sangre y colera, hazer los effectos q̃ agora acabamos d̃ declarar, assi traen consigo otra falta no pequeña, y es

Figures 4.2a and 4.2b. On the left, the title page of the 1569 edition of Nicolás Monardes's *Historia medicinal* [Medicinal history] (1565) featuring a portrait of the author. On the right, folio 181r of the British Library's copy of the *Primera parte de los problemas y secretos marauillosos de las Indias* [Problems and marvellous secrets of the Indies], showing one of several instances of hostile marginalia. Image of title page courtesy of the John Carter Brown Library. Image of fol. 181r used by permission of the British Library.

knowledge produced in the New World finding itself displaced that a new mode of colonial enunciation would arise in print. This intellectual voice, clearly discernible in the medical literature of New Spain, spoke globally to any and all 'interested readers of vernaculars' or 'curiosos romancistas', as Cárdenas called them expanding the semantic range beyond the figure of the romance surgeon, still conceiving of the Spanish *nación* as a single entity, but increasingly forced to come to terms with the trappings of coloniality and its mechanisms for marginalisation.

pests he was certain they gave rise to. For information on Camarena and his role in backing alum mining initiatives in late sixteenth-century Andalusia, see Muñoz Buendía (2007, 470–80).

Conclusion

Medical texts written about the New World during the second half of the sixteenth century are an exceptional tool with which to understand the political and cultural transformations experienced in the expanding Hispanic empire moving into the baroque era. Unlike the accounts of first explorers, which sought to amaze audiences in Europe with descriptions of strange and astonishing lands, these later texts paradoxically engaged the marvellous by stressing the need to supersede it through sustained investigation. This kind of medical writing, because of its liminal status, its use of Spanish rather than Latin, and the specific constraints of its subject matter, functioned as an unlikely early platform for a new form of regionally anchored discourse that demanded participation in a global intellectual conversation, but found itself increasingly relegated to the margins. In responding to that challenge, anatomical treatises, surgical manuals and natural histories exceeded the bounds set by European templates becoming rich, hybrid narratives that seemed just as concerned with science as they were with portraying the lives of the women and men of early modern Mexico. By examining these texts in the context of the history of science but with the tools of cultural studies and literary analysis, a new and more nuanced image of the colonial subject comes into view.

In addition to their common preoccupation with health and medicine, the more significant connection between the texts examined in *Marvels of Medicine* is not thematic but experiential. These books were different things to different readers: lifelines to essential treatment if one lived in more remote regions and could not easily fetch a surgeon; resources that enabled one to privately take care of minor, perhaps embarrassing, health problems; tools that empowered one to gauge more effectively a young and newly arrived doctor's recommended course of action; reference guides that promised a trustworthy assessment of the local foods and medicines seen in Aztec *tianguis* (regularly occurring, open-air markets[1]); rare self-portraits of your neighbours and local surroundings that felt more relevant than the representations in books

1 According to Barbara Mundy, the *tianguis* of Mexico were a 'commercial hub' as well as 'the mainstay of economic life of the city's indigenous people' (2015, 88).

arriving from Europe; gateways to formerly arcane knowledge now explained in a familiar language and available for sale in book form, outside a university space that did not welcome members of your sex; or, in some cases, windows into faraway places teeming with plants and natural phenomena you were unlikely to ever see first-hand. New Spain's reader-facing, elite yet mass-oriented medical literature brings to light information about a panoply of emerging early modern and colonial sensibilities given the ways it tried to relate to an audience. From an authorial point of view, these texts are also the testimonies of men not born colonial subjects, but who became so by virtue of how they came to understand their roles in New Spain's budding society, either as long-term or permanent residents, and through the kinds of queries science led them to formulate, which anticipated future challenges to European hegemony.

The interest shown by Benavides, Hinojosos, Farfán and Cárdenas on questions of health and science is an obvious point of contact between them, despite the many ways in which their projects differed from one another in scope and form. And yet, if we consider each writer's investment in both the scientific and social capital of early colonial Mexico, a deeper connection emerges, one that reveals their texts to be matrixes of 'colonial rhetoric' more broadly, a phenomenon Yolanda Martínez-San Miguel defines as 'a set of discursive practices that are vital in the process of constructing a colonial perspective' (2008, 27). Their texts posed some of the very same questions on epistemology, authority and identity then being raised in other discursive arenas and, while their works may be read in the context of the history of science with considerable gains, they are just as rich, if not more so, when opened to alternate avenues of critical engagement, or placed in dialogue with the wider catalogue of early colonial texts and sources. The previous chapters are all attempts to highlight more or less sequentially different elements of what is, in the end, a common story, one about the emergence of a new sense of self in relation to a place and time—New Spain in the second half of the sixteenth century—, which medical texts told in ways that are distinct but not exclusive to them in the broader context of colonial era literature and modes of cultural expression.

There is evidence to support that some of these sixteenth-century medical books continued to be of interest to readers, at least in the early part of the seventeenth century; Dorantes's and Ximénez's respective rewritings of Cárdenas are one example (see chapter 4), and the publication of a third, posthumous, edition of Farfán's *Tractado* in 1610 with news of the text being bought and sold as late as 1628 would be another.[2] But these instances notwithstanding, a compelling case cannot be made for any one of them to have had a major impact in subsequent medical practice, or to have become

2 The 'farfan de medicina' is mentioned by seventeenth-century bookseller Bartolomé de Mata in an inventory he prepared for the Inquisition of books he had acquired after 1628 (García, 2017, 54).

particularly important sources in later scientific writing. This fate is somewhat unsurprising in light of their subject matter. Works on medicine and surgery published in Europe moving into the Enlightenment tended to have a limited shelf life as newer insights superseded earlier findings, and New Spain in this regard was no different. Case in point, in his 1607 *Verdadera medicina, cirvgia y astrologia en tres libros dividida* [The true medicine, surgery and astrology divided into three books], the first new medical text printed in seventeenth-century Mexico, Juan de Barrios did mention Farfán but only to dismiss him, challenging the image his text presents of a particularly empathetic practitioner in touch with the needs of his community. Displaying what Bjørn Okholm Skaarup characterises as 'a fervent antipathy for his recently deceased colleague' Barrios instead portrayed Farfán 'as a thoroughly incompetent and indifferent medical doctor, whose patients were often saved only through Barrios' own last-minute interventions' (2015, 223). Even a source as wildly popular as Monardes's *Historia medicinal*, disseminated all over Europe, amply cited and translated into multiple languages in its day, would too be all but forgotten until the latter part of the twentieth century.

Were early colonial medical books 'thumbed out of existence in remote medical workshops', as Skaarup suggests may have happened to sources like Hinojosos's *Svmma* (2015, 214)? Perhaps. Without additional intertextual references coming to light, and with limited information on the provenance of known copies, whose very survival and good condition arguably make them the least representative specimens of their cohort, the trail of readers beyond the sixteenth century runs cold. But the significance of vernacular medical texts in a genealogy of Spanish American literature and culture is not philological but rather phenomenological. Their existence attests to how during a brief period in the sixteenth century, and using print as a vehicle, medicine claimed purchase over literacy in the Americas and the right not just to consume knowledge but to actively participate in its production, a collective gesture with far-reaching implications for the intellectual history of the region. Like fellow sixteenth-century author Bernal Díaz del Castillo, the medical writers of these works insisted theirs was the 'true' platform from which to speak about New World nature and peoples, in opposition to competing accounts assembled from afar that to them ranged in quality, from incomplete, to inexact to woefully distorted. Occupying different positions in the spectrum of early colonial medicine but brought together by common interests and by the will to take up the pen in addition to their work as health practitioners, the figures discussed in the previous chapters helped to secure the moorings of the *other* 'lettered cities' of the New World, the alternate spaces of literacy cultivated by non-elite communities of readers who would play a salient role in the rise of a distinct Latin American consciousness.[3]

3 An allusion to Ángel Rama's concept of 'the lettered city' by which he referred to the links between lettered culture and colonial institutions that policed hierarchies of power in the Americas prior to independence. For work challenging a narrow

The study of the region's literary and cultural history is still coming to terms with the breadth of representations in its millennial past, making even more pressing the need to articulate new methodological structures that enable a serious critical evaluation of materials like medical literature, formerly seen as being beyond consideration from narrow disciplinary standpoints.

definition of lettered culture and literacy in a Hispanic colonial context, see Boone and Mignolo (eds.), *Writing Without Words* (1994); Joanne Rappaport and Tom Cummins, *Beyond the Lettered City* (2011); and Jorge Cañizares-Esguerra, 'Crushing the Lettered City' (2016).

Epilogue

> 'Se conjetura que este *brave new world* es obra de una sociedad secreta de astrónomos, de biólogos, de ingenieros, de metafísicos, de poetas, de químicos, de algebristas, de moralistas, de pintores, de geómetras ...'[1]
>
> 'Tlön, Uqbar, Orbis Tertius', Jorge Luis Borges

From the very first years of European presence in the Americas, Spanish authorities attempted to limit the overseas circulation of literary texts. Referring to books of chivalry, Carlos Alberto González Sánchez summarises the crux of the Crown's initial apprehension:

> [While] in Spain, these texts were not the object of active persecution, in spite of the condemnation of the queen, of moralists, and of intellectuals ... every possible effort was made to prevent their arrival in America. The authorities felt that overseas they would endanger the supreme authority of the Bible and, therefore, the incipient evangelization of the Indians, allegedly persons of weak awareness and incapable of distinguishing between fiction and revelation ... if the missionaries demanded blind faith in equally fantastical biblical passages ... literary invention might thus become a dangerous rival to supernatural portents, those expressing the power of God and the Holy Scriptures. (2011, 60)

Edicts and ordinances would be issued repeatedly throughout the colonial era, widening the interpretation of that initial stance so as to include texts deemed 'profane' or 'frivolous' and, as discussed in the introduction, the proportional distribution by subject matter of imprints in New Spain during the sixteenth century reflects this directive, with little to nothing in the way of *romances*, or poetry, or secular works of theatre. In the Spanish case, as Martin Nesvig notes, the Crown's efforts to ban the export of the 'hugely

1 'It is conjectured that this *brave new world* is the work of a secret society comprised of astronomers, biologists, engineers, metaphysicians, poets, chemists, algebraists, moralists, painters, geometers ...', Borges (1995, 20).

popular "libros de cabellería" … or generically titled "romanceros" [were] a colossal failure' (2006, 31–32). Try as they may, on this point, orders were all too often ignored; 'papel mojado' [wet paper] the colonists would say imbuing the Atlantic with a sardonic metaphoric charge, an inescapable medium whose waters diluted and dissolved Spain's reach overseas. The inefficacy of these measures is attested by the frequency with which library inventories all over Spanish America listed imported *romances*, picaresque novels, pastorals, *comedias* and popular plays. 'Inquisitorial officials', observes Teodoro Hampe Martínez, 'were especially strict in their control of all "heretical" material, of texts that deviated from Catholic orthodoxy, but they remained relatively tolerant of others, including political and literary texts deemed "harmful" by the Crown' (2010, 63). A comparison with Portuguese America provides a sobering reminder of what was at stake. 'Quite the opposite happened in the Portuguese colonies', notes González Sánchez, 'where there were no universities, and, until the eighteenth century, books were scarce—hardly any were printed. … in 1747 the Jesuits set up a press [but it] was later dismantled by the authorities' (2011, 57). The long-standing absence of both a printing press and institutions of higher learning charted a different path toward independence for Brazil compared to the New England colonies or to territories in Spanish America that had access to resources enabling more effective political mobilisation.

To be sure, not all print was treated the same in Spanish America either, and the censorship of materials that were seen as posing a threat to Catholicism was not a minor consideration. Pedro Ocharte, the printer of both Cárdenas's *Problemas y secretos* and of the second edition of Farfán's *Tractado* would come to know this only too well, after being arrested in 1572 by the Holy Office, tortured, and having to wait two years for his release. Yet by making the reading of banned literary imports like fiction and *romances* a relatively commonplace, less transgressive infraction in Spanish America, and through the accumulation of these small acts of defiance throughout the sixteenth and seventeenth centuries, colonial societies ultimately mounted a formidable defence that secured a place for literature in a part of the world that was not supposed to have its own. At a time when the exact path events would follow on a continental scale had not yet come into focus (Lima's first book would only be published in 1584 by Antonio Ricardo, the printer who had been in charge of both Hinojosos's and Farfán's first editions), the texts written in Mexico in the sixteenth century, including the medical books by Hinojosos, Farfán and Cárdenas, helped to ensure that not all the printed material New Spain's readers held in their hands came from abroad, and that the notion of a local writer was not the exception.

Alongside medical information, the texts examined in *Marvels of Medicine* provide one of the earliest representational mirrors local readers would have, with frequent references to their own political and religious figures, recognisable geographic landmarks and a repertoire of current events relevant to them, all this achieved with the literary tools that connected reader to text.

To state that historical writing did the work of fiction in the accounts written by explorers of the so-called 'encounter' period surprises no one familiar with the history of 'marvellous-real' aesthetics in Latin American cultural studies. It is Alejo Carpentier's appeal in the last line of his prologue to *El reino de este mundo* [The Kingdom of This World] (1949); for in the end, he asks, 'what is the history of all of America if not a chronicle of the marvellous-real?'.[2] It is a claim seconded, appropriated and expanded by many other writers from the region, and given maximum exposure when embraced by leading 'Boom' writers such as Gabriel García Márquez and Carlos Fuentes.[3] The rhetorical richness of a text like Bartolomé de las Casas's *Brevísima relación de la destruición de las Indias* [An account, much abbreviated, of the destruction of the Indies] (1552), which deployed a veritable arsenal of literary tropes in an effort to persuade readers to his cause, demands the tools of literary studies in order to be fully appraised. However, the adherence to and over-identification with a masculinised imaginary closely linked to military and proselytising agendas in the literary histories of Latin America turn to a repeating subset of colonial historiography at the expense of a more diverse survey of texts and cultural objects, of which works on science and medicine are but one possible alternative itinerary.

As we have seen over the course of the preceding chapters, it was not uncommon for narrative concerns to overtake other considerations in New World medical texts. A discussion on Galen's aphorisms and Ibn Sina's surgical advice for tending to fresh wounds could be easily interrupted to remark on the limits of medicine and what doctors were and were not able to do for their patients. 'I cured a young man in Mexico using this method', writes Farfán, 'after his liver had been punctured with a sword from one side to the other ... and it was God's will that he healed to live two more years, dying a good death, having confessed his sins, since in the end he was hanged, seeing as he was incorrigible'.[4] For his part Benavides, digressing to share with his readers an example of the highly effective medicinal properties of *tunas*, told the story of 'a gentleman in the Indies by the name of Ángel de Villasaña' who quite enjoyed playing tricks on newly arrived doctors.[5]

2 '¿Pero qué es la historia de América toda sino una crónica de lo real maravilloso?' (Carpentier, 2004, 8).

3 See García Márquez's 1982 Nobel Prize speech, 'La soledad de América Latina' [The solitude of Latin America] where he claimed the 'seeds' of the Latin American novel were found in sixteenth-century explorers' accounts, as well as Fuentes's collected lectures given at Harvard University in the late 1980s, later published as *El espejo enterrado* [The buried mirror] (2010).

4 'curé en México a un mozo al cual de una estocada le pasaron de parte a parte por el hígado … y quiso Dios que sanase para que habiendo pasado dos años muriese bien, confesando sus pecados, porque le ahorcaron por incorregible' (1579, 121r).

5 'Un caballero hay en las Indias que se llama Ángel de Villasaña, que es muy donoso, y hace muchas burlas a médicos nuevos que van de esta tierra' (1567, fol. 46r).

'In his possession', explained the author, 'are always some bean powders that he has his servants put in the meals of a dinner guest, that no sooner does he finish eating he is forced to unlace his trousers, as the urgency is such, that there is no alternative.'[6] Benavides recalls an episode involving a certain Dominican friar who had been invited to supper by Villasaña and, forewarned of the man's peverse sense of humour, had managed 'very carefully and with skilful distraction' to switch his meal service undetected.[7] Despite the friar's second thoughts at seeing his host eat voraciously in an effort to get him to do the same, 'the secret did not last very long' with the man being forced to 'abandon the table and not be able to return', falling so ill 'that the aforementioned Villasaña almost died'.[8] At this point the *Secretos* returns to the topic of *tunas* and explains to the amused but likely disoriented reader the scientific relevance of the bawdy story just shared: *tunas*, even in pulverised form and mixed with water, will still have a healing effect, should you find yourself in need of treating a patient so sick with diarrhoea that he or she is unable to consume solid food, like Villasaña after his trick backfired. But which 'bean' has had such toxic effects on the body, could wonder the surgeon or doctor holding Benavides's book, eager to satisfy his professional curiosity from a medical standpoint? The text does not say. The reader is told instead that once the man had fully recovered, this scatological anecdote became a recurrent topic of conversation between Villasaña and none other than the viceroy of New Spain, Don Luis de Velasco. Velasco would taunt his friend by asking if he planned to carry on with his prankster ways after his brush with death, to which the latter would answer that he did not intend to stop until he finally succeeded in fooling a Dominican friar with his prized bean powders and thus have his revenge. 'I do not know if he has managed it yet', ends Benavides moving on to discuss a different matter, 'because I have since left [New Spain].'[9]

Readers today who come to these early colonial materials with preconceived ideas on what ought to be part of a period surgical treatise or an anatomical compendium may find themselves having to adjust their expectations. Some elements will be familiar, as they address many of the same issues that interested their European counterparts. But there will be some obvious differences. They lag behind technologically, their visual content rather underwhelming if the benchmarks in mind are Vesalius's meticulously

6 'está siempre prevenido de unos polvos de habas que hace echar en el potaje del convidado, que no ha bien acabado de comer, cuando tiene necessidad de desencintar las calzas, porque la prisa es tanta, que no tiene remedio' (1567, fol. 46v).

7 'muy disimuladamente, por vía de comedimiento pasó su seruicio al caballero sin que lo viese, y tomó el que le había servido' (1567, fol. 47r).

8 'no duró mucho el secreto, porque la prisa fue tanta, que el Ángel desamparó la mesa, y no pudo volver ... fue la burla tal que llegó Villasaña a punto de muerte' (1567, fols. 47r–47v).

9 'no sé si lo ha hecho (como lo decía) porque yo me partí' (1567, fol. 48r).

detailed flayed cadavers or Paré's fanciful prodigies and monsters—if there happen to be any images at all. What is more, these texts digress, sometimes to a fault, and it is not uncommon to come across chapters where heading and contents may bear little relation to one another. In turn, these digressions tend not to be about medical matters but feature everything from personal experiences, to conversations held with others, meditations on happiness or friendship, racist opinions, general life advice, jokes, even gossip. Case in point, before being allowed to proceed on to the medical information in Farfán's *Tractado* (1592) readers are first presented with three sonnets: two by a friend of the author, Fernán Gonçales de Eslava, and one by Farfán himself in which he dedicates the book to viceroy Velasco.[10] In the second of Eslava's poems, Farfán is turned into a character discussed by the poetic voice who holds a conversation with the allegorical figure of Illness. The poet asks:

> ¿Do vas enfermedad: *Voy desterrada.*
> ¿Quién pudo contra ti dar tal sentencia?
> *El gran doctor Farfán con pura ciencia*
> *en quien virtud del cielo está encerrada.*
> ¿Do queda la salud? *Triunfando honrada.*
> ¿De quién pudo triunfar? *De la dolencia.*
> ¿De un fraile vas huyendo? *En su presencia*
> *mi fuerza y mi poder no valen nada.*
> ¿Adónde quieres ir? *A reino extraño.*
> Allá te ofenderán los que te vieren
> que en todas partes hay también doctores.
> *Farfán solo me causa el mal y el daño*
> *pues cuantos de su libro se valieren*
> *de vida y de salud le son deudores.*
>
> [Where are you going, Illness? *I am exiled.*
> Who accomplished this?
> *The great doctor Farfán, with pure science*
> *that holds divine virtue.*
> Where is Good Health? *Justly victorious.*
> Whom did she defeat? *Sickness.*
> You flee from a friar? *In his presence*
> *my strength and my power are worthless.*
> Where would you go? *To an unknown kingdom.*
> But you will also be attacked by those who see you,
> for there are doctors in every land.
> *Farfán is the only one that harms me*

10 Farfán refers to Luis de Velasco, *hijo*, viceroy of New Spain and Peru, and the son of the one mentioned by Benavides, who had been region's second viceroy.

for any and all who turn to his book
owe him their lives and their good health.]

The personalised sonnets in this second edition of the *Tractado*, which were even more developed than the poems that had also been given a place in the first one, are another way in which a text focused on 'medicine and all the illnesses commonly encountered', if we go by its title, repeatedly gestures toward the literary and lends itself to multiple readings.[11]

At a formal level, the tropes, situations and narrative strategies present in early colonial medical sources surface in unexpected fora during the following century. One such example comes to light in a passage of a well-known source describing the medicinal properties of the Andean *matecllu* herb. In that text, its author writes:

> I used it on a boy who looked as if his eye were about to jump out of its socket. It was swollen like a pepper, the white of the eye indistinguishable from the black, being all one flesh, and it was half fallen on his cheek and the first night that I applied the herb, the eye was restored to its proper place and the second, he was completely healed. I have since seen this young man here in Spain and he has told me that he sees better out of that eye that was afflicted than out of his other one.[12]

The claims made about the health benefits of the herb are touted as exceptionally noteworthy, and aim to impress upon readers the value of a New World medicinal product like *matecllu*. However, the arrangement of the prose itself is anything but new, reminiscent of the case of Benavides's young patient with the fractured skull (discussed in chapter 1), or indeed any number of surgical treatises. *Matecllu* might have been a new element, but the rest would have seemed standard fare to a reader in 1609. First, the text dramatically establishes the seriousness of the emergency, which justifies an intervention despite grim expectations about the likelihood of success, lacking the endorsement of a doctor proper. Graphic similes elucidate the altered state of the boy's body part, followed by a suspenseful narration of the treatment undertaken. Resolution comes in the form of a wholly positive outcome—always positive, as *matasanos*, like barbarians, remain at the gates of medical texts, and failed cures are blamed on other doctors or on stubborn patients. And lastly, there is the anecdotal and enthusiastic

11 A similar point is made by Cortés Guadarrama in the introduction to his recent edition of selections from the *Tractado*, noticing the importance of the 'literary paradigms' underpinning scientific considerations for Farfán (2020, 15).

12 'Yo se la puse a un muchacho que tenía un ojo para saltarle del casco. Estaba inflamado como un pimiento, sin divisarse lo blanco ni prieto del ojo, sino hecho una carne, y lo tenía ya medio caído sobre el carrillo, y la primera noche que le puse la yerba se restituyó el ojo a su lugar y la segunda quedó del todo sano y bueno. Después acá he visto el mozo en España y me ha dicho que ve más de aquel ojo que tuvo enfermo que del otro' (Inca Garcilaso de la Vega, 2003, 150).

testimony of the procedure's lasting success, phrased, as it tends to be, in a witty fashion. This passage on American *materia medica* might not deserve any special consideration whatsoever were it not for being found inside the pages of Inca Garcilaso de la Vega's *Comentarios reales de los Incas* [Royal commentaries of the Incas] (1609), today one of the cornerstone texts in the Latin American literature canon.

The presence of scientific books in Inca Garcilaso's library has been known for some time,[13] but the extent to which these sources informed his thought process in the drafting of the *Comentarios* has not generally been a salient area of study. The work of Luis Millones Figueroa and Ronald Surtz has shed light on the text's relationship to natural history, and has shown how the treatment of autochthonous flora and fauna compared against the way imported European crops and animals were portrayed amounted to a critique of power imbalance in early colonial society.[14] But it is only recently that the links to medicine and physiology are being scrutinised more closely, from moments when the *Comentarios* directly gloss Monardes,[15] to the author's refashioning of terminology like 'mestizo' and 'cuatralbo', first found in European treatises on botany and veterinary medicine [*albeitería*] theorising emerging New World racial categories, as Ruth Hill's research has uncovered.[16] In Inca Garcilaso's world, which at the time of drafting the *Comentarios* was Spain in the midst of a literary Golden Age, allusions to illness and to medical treatments abounded. They informed plot lines in plays like Lope de Vega's *El acero de Madrid* [The steel of Madrid] (1608) and Pedro Calderón de la Barca's *El médico de su honra* [The physician of his honour] (1637). They lent their terminology to picaresque prose as in Mateo Alemán's *El Guzmán de Alfarache* [The rouge: or the life of Guzman de Alfarache] (1599),[17] and medical books were placed also in the hands

13 Although his efforts have since been updated, already in 1948 José Durand listed the contents of the author's library as found in documentary evidence and speculated on the identities of titles with more than one possible authorial attribution. See Durand, 'La biblioteca del Inca'. The subject was recently revisited in the catalogue of the Biblioteca Nacional de España's 2016 exhibition 'La biblioteca del Inca Garcilaso de la Vega', which includes a commentary of a selection of works, including Monardes's *Historia*, by Esperanza López Parada, Marta Ortiz Canseco and Paul Firbas, as well as a facsimile and a transcript of the books listed in the author's possession upon his death.

14 See Millones Figueroa (2009) and Surtz (2014).

15 For the intertextual connection between Inca Garcilaso and Monardes, see Pérez Marín, 2015.

16 For a discussion on the author's use of concepts explored in sixteenth-century botany and veterinary medicine, especially horse-breeding, see Hill, 2015, 45–64.

17 As Francisco Ramírez Santacruz remarks, 'for Alemán the world is inhabited by men of corrupt reasoning whose vices are manifested pathologically. This worldview has a linguistic correspondence. Fevers [calenturas], pox [sarampión], lesions [ciciones], vomit [vómito], drowsiness [modorra] are words consistently repeated throughout the novel, where there is a vast system of images based on human anatomy and pharmacy'

of characters like Sabuco's unlikely shepherds (see chapter 4) who debated the finer points of Monardes's *Historia medicinal*. Possibly the most famous self-professed period 'reader' of medical books is Don Quixote who, after an unfortunate encounter with ewes and sheep that leave him and his squire battered and famished, concedes that he would have preferred 'a quarter of bread, or a loaf and two pilchards' heads to all the herbs described by Dioscorides, even if it were the one illustrated by doctor Laguna', a quietly elegant acknowledgement on Cervantes's part of Andrés Laguna's publication from 50 years before.[18]

Cervantes was not alone in using medical books in artistic endeavours to tell us more about a represented subject's intellectual sensibilities. Sor Juana Inés de la Cruz, who along with Inca Garcilaso, is a defining voice in the cultural and literary history of Latin America, displayed in her writings a level of mastery over European learned culture superior to that of most educated *criollos* of her time, male or female. But, as noted by Juan Castro, the gaps in her education are just as telling: 'Octavio Paz's reconstruction of Sor Juana's library gives a clear image of the intellectual isolation of the Spanish colonial world. Sor Juana had a large personal library—between 1,500, the number estimated by Paz, and 4,000 books, the number given by her original biographer Diego Calleja in 1700' (2008, 11). And yet, despite its size, Paz found that '"the new science and the new political philosophy [were] not represented"' (cited in Castro, 2008, 11). Some of Sor Juana's most noted literary conversations were with sources written well before her time. António Vieira's *Sermão do mandato* [Maundy Thursday Sermon] was delivered mid century in Lisbon around the same time sor Juana was born, later becoming the subject of the critique she advanced in the 'Carta atenagórica' [Letter worthy of Athena] (1690), the unauthorised dissemination of which would prompt her to write the *Respuesta a sor Filotea de la Cruz* [Response to sor Filotea] (1691), in turn, one of the most important documents in defence of women's intellectual capacities of the early modern period. The generational gap is even more pronounced in the dialogue she posits with Góngora in lyric compositions such as 'A su retrato' [Poem 145],[19] the Spanish poet

(2005, 37). For an analysis of how Alemán's experience as a medical student at the University of Alcalá impacted his literary craft, see Ramírez Santacruz (2005). The impact of a medical-surgical sensibility on the work of key thinkers and figures in the Latin American cultural tradition, beyond the early modern period (Ramón Emeterio Betances, Baldomero Fernández Moreno, João Guimarães Rosa, Ernesto 'Che' Guevara, Salvador Allende) is a subject yet to be fully explored.

18 'un cuartal de pan, o una hogaza y dos cabezas de sardinas arenques, por cuantas yerbas describe Dioscórides, aunque fuera el ilustrado por el doctor Laguna' (1994, 181).

19 Góngora's famed sonnet CLXVI, 'Mientras por competir por tu cabello' [While to compete with your hair], containing one of the best-known examples of *gradatio* in Hispanic literature, is evoked by Sor Juana in her own poem which rewrites the

being long dead by then. A significant exception to this trend was her study of Athanasius Kircher, the Jesuit polymath who stands as a key figure in European intellectual history, and whose work provided a connection to a wider arena of scientific thought, becoming, as Paula Findlen explains, an 'inspiration for her ideas about nature, history, religion, music, optics, and astronomy' (2004, 349).

Turning not to Sor Juana's own possible intellectual dialogue with scientific or medical literature, which would be a project to its own, let us consider instead in this epilogue the connections that were imagined for her by two portraits painted after her death, the first attributed to Juan de Miranda (d. 1714) created not long after Sor Juana's passing, and the other by Miguel Cabrera (1695–1768) which dates to 1750. Both paintings show the writer at her desk against the backdrop of her private library. In Miranda's portrait, Sor Juana's connection to scientific enquiry is hard to ignore. She is shown, quill in one hand, rosary on the other, looking firmly at the viewer. But behind her is a partial view of a space in active use, with some books hurriedly filed away, their leather ties half undone, some turned on their sides to the point viewers cannot make out the titles on their spines. Among these is one on the second shelf that raises particular concern, precariously balanced on top of another, in danger of spilling the liquid-filled alchemical beaker beneath should it fall, an object that is casually pinning down a small paper note with hand-drawn geometric figures and calculations. Among the titles the viewer can clearly identify are works by Saint Augustine and Aristotle, as well as 'a book purporting to be the Opera Kirkerio' (Findlen, 2004, 334). Cabrera would also include a reference to Kircher in his own version of Sor Juana's library (see figure 5.1), which holds even more titles than Miranda's. This rendition keeps many of Miranda's elements, like the clock, but the desk is moved forward so that more of her library is visible. The change most often noted between the two famous portraits is in Sor Juana's posture, who appears seated in Cabrera's version, quill in its inkwell and captured not in the act of writing but of reading instead.[20]

Cabrera's painting is a baroque game of references open to multiple and even contradictory interpretations. On the one hand, as has been recently argued by Charlene Villaseñor Black, he offers a 'pictorial vindication' of Sor Juana by inviting the viewer to link her through formal and symbolic associations with depictions of scholars and holy women (2016, 227). But in contrast to other visual representations of academics, or portraits of court figures, where only one or two texts might be identifiable, the importance given to

last verse and would go on to become an equally famous composition in the literary canon.

20 For a study of Sor Juana's portraits, see Villaseñor Black, 'Portraits of Sor Juana Inés de la Cruz and the Dangers of Intellectual Desire'. Villaseñor Black leaves open the possibility that Cabrera worked from a lost original, but names Miranda's painting as a probable source (2016, 216).

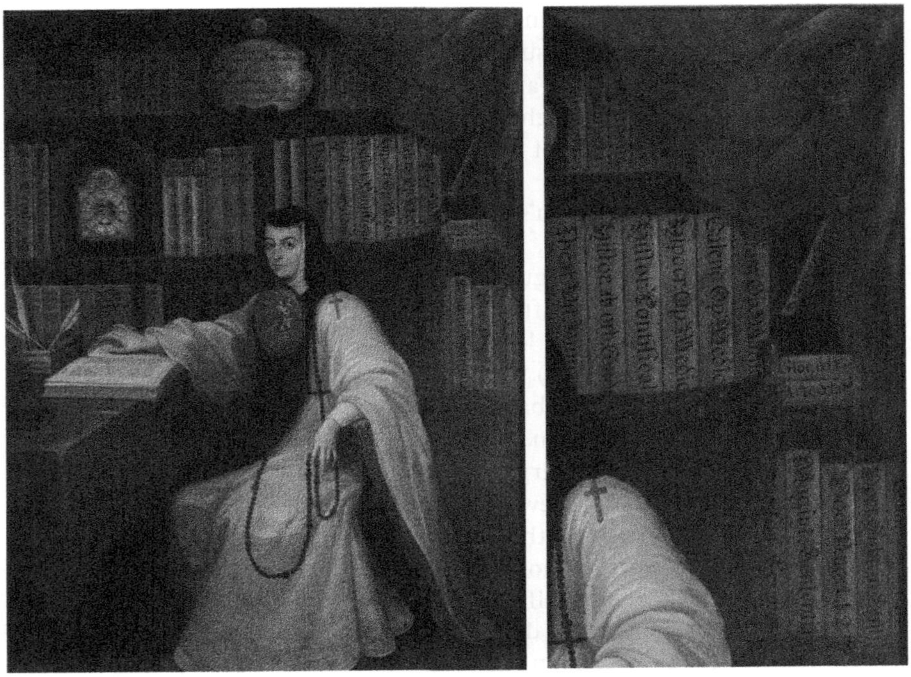

Figure 5.1. Posthumous portrait of Sor Juana Inés de la Cruz in her private cell by Miguel Cabrera, (1750), oil on canvas (left). Detail of the same (right) showing in the middle shelf works by Galen, Hippocrates, Kircher and possibly Beyerlinck. Quarto-sized tomes in the upper shelf are identified as 'Chirurgia', 'Pharmacia' and 'Anatomia' next to a partial view of a fourth labelled 'Gongora', and a fifth that possibly reads '[Marco] Polo'. Reproduction authorised by the Instituto Nacional de Antropología e Historia, Mexico City, Mexico.

the titles in her collection is striking. Only a few books are either obscured by shadow or by the requisite red curtain present in so many colonial era portraits with the identities of the rest on display for the viewer to take note. According to Findlen, there is a coded message in both paintings that underscores the relationship between Sor Juana and science using Kircher as its fulcrum. In Miranda's portrait, the 'Opera Kirkerio' is 'shoved into a corner' behind Sor Juana's own texts (Findlen, 2004, 334). In Cabrera's portrait, the renamed 'Kirqueri Opera' is present as well, but is further condensed visually, becoming the slimmest of all the titles in the background. Sor Juana's copies of Kircher, explains Findlen:

> were of course more than one book. In their entirety, a total of fifty-four printed volumes and some thirty books, they would have filled her imaginary library. Both Miranda and Cabrera—who knew something

> about the material appearance of these books and expected their viewers to get the joke—reduced some of the largest, most numerous, and weighty volumes ever to fill the shelves of any library down to a slim, inconsequential tome, just as Sor Juana condensed Kircher's ideas in her poems, transforming his prolix Latin sentences into short, elegant Castilian phrases. (2004, 335)

Findlen's observation on this point and her interpretation become even more plausible when we realise the gesture is repeated with another text shown in both portraits. Present, but compressed as well among Latin versions of Hippocrates and Galen in Cabrera's painting is possibly Laurens Beyerlinck's *Magnum Theatrum Vitae Humanae* which ran into the thousands of pages.[21] But if monumental texts and emerging encyclopaedic projects stand reduced, what is then amplified in the painting's visual space in relation to them?

Resting on the top right-hand shelf, the most likely of all the books to be hidden from the viewer should the ties of the curtain on the right become loose, are three quarto-sized books whose spines read 'Chirurgia', 'Pharmacia' and 'Anathomia', filed adjacent to a partially obscured fourth where the reader can scarcely make out the word 'Gongora'. Cabrera gives his audience just enough information to make it wonder if it is indeed the famed poet in light of the known intertexual relationship between him and Sor Juana. In the context of the games already being played in the library, one possible interpretation is that this is yet another joke, this time at Góngora's expense, having one of the paradigmatic figures of the Hispanic baroque being pushed into a corner by books viewers would deem of much lesser artistic quality and considerably lower literary remit; indeed, not just Góngora but Marco Polo's *Travels*, the last partially visible tome on the shelf and a key source of inspiration for Columbus, is also given the same treatment. And yet the presence of medical books next to one of Sor Juana's most important influences and close to another that had so fuelled Europe's imagination in its project of global expansion also raises

21 According to Francisco de la Maza, this title is indeed Laurens Beyerlinck's *Magnum Theatrum Vitae Humanae*, first published in Cologne in 1631 in seven volumes and expanded into eight in subsequent editions (1980, 303); Elías Trabulse confirms that Beyerlinck circulated in Mexico, explaining that information cited by Sor Juana's contemporary, Carlos de Sigüenza y Góngora, could only have been known through access to this text (1994, 154–55). It should be noted, however, that Beyerlink's work is 'in fact a reworked and carefully purged edition of the *Theatrum vitae humanae* [written by] Protestant physician Theodorus Zwinger' (Houdt, 2000, 107). Zwinger's text, published in 1565 is considered 'perhaps the world's largest single collection of commonplace excerpts ... running to over 5,000 double-column folio pages of small type" (Ong, 1976, 111). Cabrera's illustration does not include the word 'Magnum', introducing a small chance the reference is to Zwinger's rather than to Beyerlinck's shorter yet still voluminous *Theatrum*.

them by association, serving as reminders of her standing as a New World polymath.[22]

Books and print culture were important for Cabrera. Although today he is remembered primarily as a painter and major figure in the history Latin American visual culture for his work on portraiture and his casta series, he is also the author of a short treatise called the *Maravilla americana y conjunto de raras maravillas* [American marvel and collection of rare marvels] published in Mexico in 1756. In the *Maravilla,* Cabrera expanded on a report he had written after being called along with seven other painters to examine the then over 200-year-old sacred image of Our Lady of Guadalupe in order to issue an opinion as to whether it was a work of divine or human creation; Cabrera would support the view that it was indeed the work of angels rather than men. His analysis considered the painting both as a material and as an artistic object, and commented on matters such as the likely provenance of the canvas and pigments as well as the stylistic composition. In a section where he explains why he preferred using an older unit of measurement to describe the proportions of the human body in the painting's artistic space, Cabrera writes:

> And let no one be surprised that we measure this image by *rostros* rather than modules, as that was the practice of the princes of this discipline, Apelles, Phidias, Lysippos; and our own Spaniards Juan de Arce and Gaspar Becerra, that there has always been variety in the order of the numbers of *rostros* or sizes of the human body, as some divided it by ten, others by nine and a half and a third, and others by nine.[23]

The fame of Apelles of Kos and Lysippos has withstood the test of time, but Becerra is perhaps more challenging to place for the modern reader, even if it is likely that he or she has come across his work by way of the famous image

22 While true that images of reading men 'seated at their desks surrounded by books' are a trope almost exclusively reserved for men in paintings, as Villaseñor Black observes (222), there are precedents of female sitters in European manuscript and print culture illustrations. John Sturt's frontispiece for Theophilus Dorrington's *The Excellent Woman Described by Her True Characters and Their Opposites* (London: Joseph Watts, 1692), an English translation of Jacques du Bosc's *L'Honneste femme, divisée en trois parties* (1632–36), like Cabrera's portrait of Sor Juana, shows a woman sitting at her desk, with a bookcase in the background divided into the areas of 'Divinity', 'Morality', 'History', 'Poetry', 'Physick' and 'Surgery' (see 'The Excellent Woman' in the 'Gallery' section of the portal she-philosopher.com). I am indebted to independent scholar Deborah Taylor-Pearce, editor of this web-based research project, for her guidance on this matter and for bringing to my attention the existence of this engraving.

23 'Y no se extrañe este modo de mesurar nuestra imagen por rostros, y no por módulos: que así lo practicaron los príncipes de esta facultad, como fueron Apeles, Fidias y Lisipo; y de nuestros españoles Juan de Arce y Gaspar Becerra: bien, que siempre ha habido variedad en orden al número de rostros, o tamaños de el cuerpo humano: porque unos lo regularon por diez, otros por nueve y medio, y un tercio, y otros por nueve' (1756, 7).

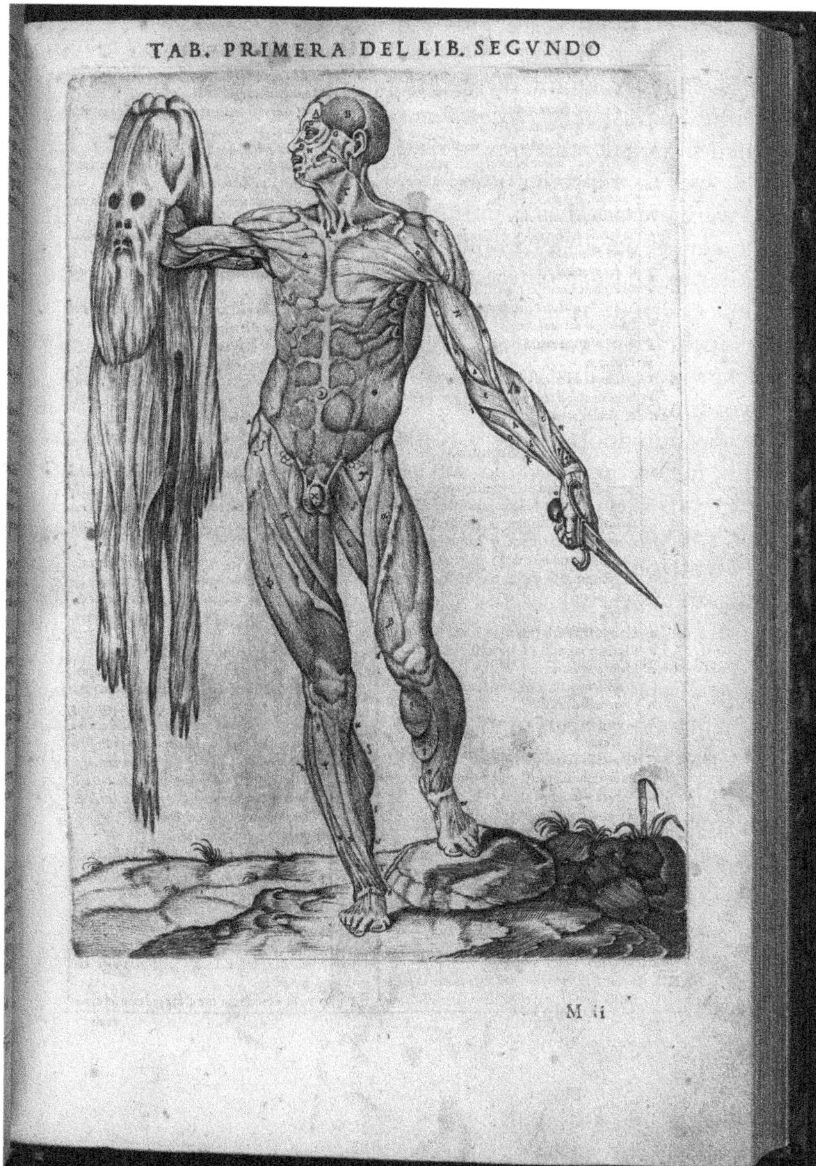

Figure 5.2. Image accompanying the first table in book two of Juan Valverde de Amusco's first edition of the *Historia de la composición del cuerpo humano* [Anatomy of the human body] (Rome, 1556). Valverde famously copied many of Vesalius's illustrations from the *Fabrica* (Padua, 1543) in his own text, which the latter denounced, but the image above was among the *Historia*'s new visual content. The engraving is attributed to Nicolas Béatrizet, based on a drawing by Gaspar Becerra, the artistic master adduced by Cabrera. Used by permission of the British Library.

of 'the flayed man holding his own skin' (see figure 5.2), one of the engravings attributed to him in Juan Valverde de Amusco's *Historia de la composición del cuerpo humano* [Anatomy of the human body] (1556). Published in Rome and written in Spanish, the *Historia de la composición* quickly became a widely disseminated source on anatomy in its day. Classical and European templates, originals as well as reproductions, were part of the artistic capital of New Spain and were imported as commodities, so it is possible that Cabrera would have come across copies of paintings or sculptures by Becerra and that is how he came to know about his work. But the more plausible route is that the contact occurred, as it often did, by way of print, through the detailed engravings included in books on botany and medicine, like the ones he places in the background of his portrait of Sor Juana. Indeed, given the context and the wording of the passage in the *Maravilla americana* on the 'human body' [cuerpo humano], Cabrera is likely referring to the title Valverde had given to his major opus. While we lack evidence that would let us put an anatomical treatise in Sor Juana's hands, there is a strong case to be made for placing it in those of one of her portraitists, a major voice of the colonial era in his own right.

Listening more closely to the dialogue between science, medicine, print culture and artistic representation brings us a step closer to grasping the range of sensibilities and interests held by colonial subjects in the early modern period. For Cabrera, as he endeavoured to capture the reality of Sor Juana's life on canvas, and as someone deeply invested in the artistic and intellectual life of viceregal Mexico, her library would not have been complete without works on surgery and medicine. Our own literary and cultural histories of Latin America would not be either.

Works cited

Acosta, José de. *Natural and Moral History of the Indies*. Ed. Jane E. Mangan. Tr. Frances López-Morillas. Durham, NC and London: Duke UP, 2002.

Acuña-Soto, Rodolfo, D. W. Stahle, M. K. Cleaveland and M. D. Therrell. 'Megadrought and Megadeth in 16th Century Mexico'. *Emerging Infectious Diseases* 8.4 (2002): 360–62.

Adorno, Rolena. *The Polemics of Possession in Spanish American Narrative*. New Haven, CT and London: Yale UP, 2007.

Ainsworth, Claire. 'Sex redefined'. *Nature* 518.7539 (2015): 288–91.

Albarracín Teulón, Agustín. *La medicina en el teatro de Lope de Vega*. Madrid: Consejo Superior de Investigaciones Científicas, 1954.

Alcocer y Martínez, Mariano. *Catálogo razonado de obras impresas en Valladolid, 1481–1800*. Valladolid: Imprenta de la Casa Social Católica, 1926.

Álvarez Peláez, Raquel. *La conquista de la naturaleza americana*. Cuadernos Galileo de la Historia de la Ciencia. Madrid: Consejo Superior de Investigaciones Científicas, 1993.

Ambrosi, Paola and Matteo De Beni. '*Tomar el acero y pasearlo*. Notas lingüísticas y culturológicas en torno al significado médico de la voz acero'. *Quien lengua ha Roma va. Studi di Lingua e Traduzione per Carmen Navarro*. Eds. Francesca Dalle Pezze, Matteo de Beni and Renzo Miotti. Mantua: Universitas Studiorum, 2014. 37–70.

Arias de Benavides, Pedro. *Secretos de Chirurgia, especial de las enfermedades de Morbo galico y Lamparones y Mirrarchia, y assi mismo la manera como se curan los Indios de llagas y heridas y otras passiones en las Indias, muy vtil y prouechoso para en España y otros muchos secretos de chirurgia hasta agora no escriptos*. Valladolid: Francisco Fernández de Córdoba, 1567.

Balbuena, Bernardo de. *La grandeza mexicana y Compendio apologético en alabanza de la poesía*. [1604]. Mexico: Editorial Porrúa, 1997.

Ball, Catherine A. et al. 'Ethnicity Estimate 2019 White Paper'. *AncestryDNA*, www.ancestry.com/corporate/sites/default/files/AncestryDNA-Ethnicity-White-Paper.pdf.

——. 'Iberian Ethnicity'. *AncestryDNA*, www.ancestry.com/dna/ethnicity/iberian-peninsula.

Barrera-Osorio, Antonio. *Experiencing Nature: The Spanish American Empire and the Early Scientific Revolution*. Austin: U of Texas P, 2006.

Bauer, Ralph. *The Alchemy of Conquest: Science, Religion, and the Secrets of the New World*. Charlottesville and London: U of Virginia P, 2019.

——. 'The Blood of the Dragon: Alchemy and Natural History in Nicolás Monardes's Historia medicinal'. *Medical Cultures of the Early Modern Spanish Empire*. Eds. John Slater, Maríaluz López-Terrada and José Pardo Tomás. Surrey: Ashgate, 2014. 67–88.

Bauer, Ralph and José Antonio Mazzotti. 'Introduction: Creole Subjects in the Colonial Americas'. *Creole Subjects in the Colonial Americas: Empires, Texts, Identities*. Eds. Ralph Bauer and José Antonio Mazzotti. Chapel Hill: U of North Carolina P, 2009. 1–57.

Bennett, Herman L. *Africans in Colonial Mexico: Absolutism, Christianity, and Afro-Creole Consciousness, 1570–1640*. Bloomington and Indianapolis: Indiana UP, 2003.

Beusterien, John. *Canines in Cervantes and Velázquez: An Animal Studies Reading of Early Modern Spain*. London and New York: Routledge, 2016.

Bleichmar, Daniela. 'Books, Bodies, and Fields: Sixteenth-Century Transatlantic Encounters with New World *Materia Medica*'. *Colonial Botany: Science, Commerce, and Politics in the Early Modern World*. Eds. Londa Schiebinger and Claudia Swan. Philadelphia: U of Pennsylvania P, 2005. 83–99.

Blell, Mwenza and M. A. Hunter. 'Direct-to-Consumer Genetic Testing's Red Herring: "Genetic Ancestry" and Personalized Medicine'. *Frontiers in Medicine* 6.48 (2019): n. pag. www.frontiersin.org/articles/10.3389/fmed.2019.00048/full. 11 Feb. 2020.

Borges, Jorge Luis. *Ficciones*. [1944]. Madrid: Alianza Editorial, 1995.

Brading, David. *Miners and Merchants in Bourbon Mexico 1763–1810*. Digital version. Cambridge: Cambridge UP, 2008.

Brendecke, Arndt. *The Empirical Empire: Spanish Colonial Rule and the Politics of Knowledge*. Berlin: Walter de Gruyter, 2016.

Brian, Amber. 'Shifting Identities: Mestizo Historiography and the Representation of Chichimecs'. *To Be Indio in Colonial Spanish America*. Ed. Mónica Díaz. Albuquerque: U of New Mexico P, 2017. 143–66.

Brouard Uriarte, J. L. 'Médicos, cirujanos, barberos y algebristas castellanos del siglo XV'. *Cuadernos de Historia de la Medicina Española* 11 (1972): 239–53.

Bruster, Douglas and Robert Weimann. *Prologues to Shakespeare's Theater: Performance and Liminality in Early Modern Drama*. New York: Routledge, 2004.

Cabezas, Lino, Inmaculada López Vílchez, Juan Carlos Oliver, Raúl Campos López and Manuel Barbero. Eds. *Dibujo científico: arte y naturaleza, ilustración científica, infografía, esquemática*. Dibujo y profesión 4. Madrid: Cátedra, 2016.

Cabré, Monserrat. 'Keeping Beauty Secrets in Early Modern Iberia'. *Secrets and Knowledge in Medicine and Science*, 1500–1800. Eds. Elaine Leong and Alisha Rankin. Surrey: Ashgate, 2011. 167–90.

Cabrera, Miguel. *Maravilla americana y conjunto de raras maravillas*. Mexico: Imprenta del Real y mas Antiguo Colegio de San Ildefonso, 1756.

Campbell, Mary Baine. *Wonder & Science: Imagining Worlds in Early Modern Europe*. Ithaca, NY: Cornell UP, 1999.

Cañizares-Esguerra, Jorge. 'Crushing the Lettered City: Theological Worlds of the Illiterate'. University of London. School of Advanced Study, London. Inaugural LAGLOBAL/Leverhulme Trust Lecture. 4 February 2016. Lecture.

——. *How to Write the History of the New World: Histories, Epistemologies, and Identities in the Eighteenth-Century Atlantic World*. Stanford, CA: Stanford UP, 2001.

——. 'New World, New Stars: Patriotic Astrology and the Invention of Indian and Creole Bodies in Colonial Spanish America, 1600–1650'. *Nature, Empire, and Nation: Explorations of the History of Science in the Iberian World*. Stanford, CA: Stanford UP, 2006. 64–95.

——. 'Racial, Religious, and Civic Creole Identity in Colonial Spanish America'. *American Literary History* 17.3 (2005): 420–37.

Carbón, Damián. *Libro del arte delas Comadres, o madrinas, y del regimiento delas preñadas y paridas, y delos niños*. Mallorca: Hernando de Cansoles, 1541.

Cardeira, Esperança. 'Preto and negro, pardo, mestiço and mulato'. *Colour and Colour Naming: Crosslinguistic Approaches*. Eds. João Paulo Silvestre, Esperança Cardeira and Alina Villalva. Lisbon: Centro de Linguística da Universidade de Lisboa & Universidade de Aveiro, 2016. 71–87.

Cárdenas, Juan de. *Primera parte de los problemas y secretos marauillosos de las Indias*. Mexico: Pedro Ocharte, 1591.

——. *Problemas y secretos maravillosos de las Indias*. [1591]. Madrid: Alianza, 1988.

Carpentier, Alejo. *El reino de este mundo*. [1949]. San Juan: Editorial de la Universidad de Puerto Rico, 2004.

Castro, Juan E. *The Spaces of Latin American Literature: Tradition, Globalization, and Cultural Production*. New York: Palgrave MacMillan, 2008.

Cátedra, Pedro M. *Nobleza y lectura en tiempos de Felipe II: la biblioteca de Don Alonso Osorio, Marqués de Astorga*. Valladolid: Junta de Castilla y León, Consejería de Educación y Cultura, 2002.

Catholic Church. *Constituciones del arçobispado y prouincia dela muy ynsigne y muy leal ciudad de Tenuxtitlan Mexico dela nueua España*. Mexico: Juan Pablos, 1556.

Cavillac, Michel. 'La cour de Monipodio, cour des miracles'. *Séville XVIe siècle: de Colomb à don Quichotte, entre Europe et Amériques, le coeur du richesses du monde*. Ed. Carlos Martínez Shaw. Paris: Autrement, 1992. 114–30.

Cervantes, Miguel de. *El ingenioso hidalgo don Quijote de la Mancha*. Ed. Martín de Riquer. Barcelona: Editorial Planeta, 1994.

Cervantes de Salazar, Francisco. *Crónica de la Nueva España*. Ed. Manuel Magallón. Biblioteca de autores españoles. Vol. 244. Madrid: Ediciones Atlas, 1971.

Chauliac, Guy de. *Inventarium sive Chirurgia Magna*. 1363. Ed. and tr. Michael R. McVaugh. Vol. 1. Leiden: E. J. Brill, 1997.

——. 'Is Surgery a Science? (3): Guy de Chauliac's History of Surgery'. *Medieval Medicine: A Reader*. Ed. Faith Wallis. Tr. James Bruce Ross. Toronto: U of Toronto P, 2010. 296–300.

Chaves, María Eugenia. 'Beyond Race: Exclusion in Early Modern Spain and Spanish America'. *Race and Blood in the Iberian World.* Eds. Max S. Hering Torres, María Elena Martínez and David Nirenberg. Zurich, Berlin: LIT Verlag, 2012. 39–58.

Chico, Ponce de León, J. T. Goodrich, M. Tutino and C. Gordon. 'First Published Record of a Neurosurgical Procedure on the North American Continent'. *Neurosurgery* 47 (2000): 216–22.

Chinchilla, Anastacio. *Anales históricos de la medicina en general, y biográfico-bibliográfico de la española en particular.* Historia de la medicina española. Vol. 1. Valencia: Imprenta de D. López y Compañía, 1841.

Cleminson, Richard and Francisco Vázquez García. *Sex, Identity and Hermaphrodies in Iberia, 1500–1800.* London: Pickering & Chatto, 2013.

Colón, Cristóbal. 'Quarta Viage de Colón'. *Select Documents Illustrating the Four Voyages of Columbus.* Eds. Cecil Jane and E. G. R. Taylor. Vol. II. London: The Hakluyt Society, 1993. 72–111.

——. *Textos y documentos completos.* Ed. Consuelo Varela. Madrid: Alianza, 1995.

Comas, Juan. 'La influencia indígena en la medicina hipocrática en la Nueva España del siglo XVI'. *El mestizaje cultural y la medicina novohispana del siglo XVI.* Eds. J. L. Fresquet Febrer and J. M. López Piñero. Valencia: Instituto de Estudios Documentales e Históricos sobre la Ciencia, Universitat de València – CSIC, 1995. 91–127.

Conrad, Lawrence I. and Dominik Wujastyk. 'Introduction'. *Contagion: Perspectives from Pre-Modern Societies.* Eds. Lawrence I. Conrad and Dominik Wujastyk. London and New York: Routledge, 2017. ix–xviii.

Cook, Noble David. 'Disease and the depopulation of Hispaniola, 1492–1518'. *Colonial Latin American Review* 2.1–2 (1993): 213–45.

Correas, Gonzalo. *Vocabulario de refranes y frases proverbiales (1627).* Eds. Louis Combet, Robert Jammes and Maïte Mir-Andreu. Madrid: Editorial Castalia, 2000.

Covarrubias, Sebastián de. *Tesoro de la Lengua Castellana o Española.* 1611. Ed. Martín de Riquer. Barcelona: Editorial Alta Fulla, 1998.

Cruz-Sotomayor, Beatriz. '*Tan estraño y nuevo es el libro, quanto es el autor*': *autoría y recepción en la Nueva filosofía de Oliva Sabuco.* PhD dissertation. University of Puerto Rico, Río Piedras. Ann Arbor: ProQuest/UMI, 2008. (Publication No. AAT 3325861.)

Deans-Smith, Susan. 'Creating the Colonial Subject: Casta Paintings, Collectors, and Critics in Eighteenth-Century Mexico and Spain'. *Colonial Latin American Review* 14.2 (2005): 169–204.

Diccionario de Autoridades. Vol. 2. 'cientifico/ca'. Real Academia Española. 1729. https://www.rae.es/recursos/diccionarios/diccionarios-anteriores-1726-1996/diccionario-de-autoridades. 1 Aug. 2016.

Dioscorides. *Pedacio Dioscorides Anazarbeo, acerca de la materia medicinal, y de los venenos mortiferos, Traduzido de lengua Griega, en la vulgar Castellana & illustrado con claras y substantiales Annotationes, y con las figuras de innumeras plantas exquisitas y raras.* Tr. Andrés Laguna. Antwerp: Juan Latio, 1555.

Dixon, Laurinda S. *Perilous Chastity: Women and Illness in Pre-Enlightenment Art and Medicine.* Ithaca, NY: Cornell UP, 1995.

Dorrington, Theophilus. *The Excellent Woman Described by Her True Characters and Their Opposites*. London: Joseph Watts, 1692. Translation of Jacques Du Bosc, *L'Honneste femme, divisée en trois parties*. Paris: Pierre Billaine, 1632–36.

Durand, José. 'La biblioteca del Inca'. *Nueva Revista de Filología Hispánica* 2 (1948): 174–85.

Eamon, William. 'Medicine as a Hunt: Searching for the Secrets of the New World'. *Renaissance Futurities: Science, Art, Invention*. Eds. Charlene Villaseñor Black and Mari-Tere Álvarez. Oakland: U of California P, 2019. 100–17.

——. *Science and the Secrets of Nature: Books of Secrets in Medieval and Early Modern Culture*. Princeton, NJ: Princeton UP, 1994.

——. 'The charlatan's trial: an Italian surgeon in the court of King Philip II, 1576–1577'. *Cronos* 8.1 (2005): 3–30.

Earenfight, Theresa. *The King's Other Body: María of Castile and the Crown of Aragon*. Philadelphia: U of Pennsylvania P, 2010.

Earle, Rebecca. *The Body of the Conquistador: Food, Race and the Colonial Experience in Spanish America, 1492–1700*. Cambridge: Cambridge UP, 2012.

Egerton, Frank N. 'A History of the Ecological Sciences, Part 13: Broadening Science in Italy and England, 1600–1650'. *Bulletin of the Ecological Society of America* July (2004): 110–19.

Endersby, Jim. *A Guinea Pig's History of Biology*. Cambridge, MA: Harvard UP, 2007.

Enríquez, Martín de. Letter to the Council of the Indies. 18 October 1579. AGI, Mexico, 20, N.29. Manuscript.

Farfán, Agustín. *Tractado breve de anothomia y chirvgia, y de algvnas enfermedades, que mas comunmente suelen hauer en esta Nueua España*. Mexico: Antonio Ricardo, 1579.

——. *Tractado brebe de Medicina, y de todas las enfermedades*. [1592]. Colección de incunables americanos. Vol. 10. Madrid: Ediciones Cultura Hispánica, 1944.

——. *Tratado breve de medicina y de todas las enfermedades*. [1592]. Ed. Marcos Cortés Guadarrama. Madrid: Iberoamericana Vervuert, 2020.

Fausto-Sterling, Anne. *Sex/Gender: Biology in a Social World*. New York and London: Routledge, 2012.

Fernández de Enciso, Martín. *Suma de geographia que trata de todas las partidas y prouincias del mundo: en especial delas indias*. Seville: Jacobo Cromberger, 1519.

Fernández de Oviedo, Gonzalo. *Historia general y natural de Indias*. Ed. Juan Pérez de Tudela Bueso. Biblioteca de autores españoles. Vol. 117. Madrid: Ediciones Atlas, 1959.

——. *La historia general delas Indias*. Seville: Juan Cromberger, 1535.

——. *Sumario de la natural historia de las Indias*. Ed. José Miranda. 2nd printing. Mexico: Fondo de Cultura Económica, 1996.

Fernández de Zamora, Rosa María. *Los impresos mexicanos del siglo XVI: su presencia en el patrimonio cultural del nuevo siglo*. Mexico: UNAM, 2009.

Figueras Vallés, Estrella. Fray Tomás de Berlanga. *Una vida dedicada a la Fe y a la Ciencia*. Soria: Ochoa Impresores, 2010.

Findlen, Paula. 'A Jesuit's Books in the New World: Athanasius Kircher and his American Readers'. *Athanasius Kircher: The Last Man Who Knew Everything*. Ed. Paula Findlen. New York and London: Routledge, 2004. 329–64.

Foucault, Michel. *Archaeology of Knowledge*. Tr. A. M. Sheridan Smith. London and New York: Routledge, 2002.

——. *The Order of Things*. Taylor and Francis e-Library. London and New York: Routledge, 2005.

Fracchia, Carmen. *Black but Human: Slavery and Visual Art in Hapsburg Spain, 1480–1700*. Oxford: Oxford UP, 2019.

Fragoso, Juan. *Cirvgia vniversal, aora nvevamente añadida, con todas las dificvltades, y qvestiones, pertenecientes a las materias que se trata*. [1581]. Madrid: Viuda de Alonso Martin, 1627.

Fresquet Febrer, José Luis. *La experiencia americana y la terapéutica en los Secretos de Chirurgia (1567) de Pedro Arias de Benavides. Cuadernos Valencianos de Historia de la Medicina y de la Ciencia*. Vol. XLI. Valencia: Universitat de València – CSIC, 1993.

Fresquet Febrer, José Luis and María Luz López-Terrada. 'Plantas mexicanas en Europa en el siglo XVI'. *Arqueología mexicana* 39 (1999): 38–43.

Fuentes, Carlos. *El espejo enterrado. Reflexiones sobre España y América*. Madrid: Alfaguara, 2010.

García, Idalia. 'The importation of Books into New Spain During the Seventeenth Century'. *A Maturing Market: The Iberian Book World in the First Half of the Seventeenth Century*. Eds. Alexander S. Wilkinson and Alejandra Ulla Lorenzo. Leiden: Brill, 2017. 45–66.

García Ballester, Luis. *La búsqueda de la salud. Sanadores y enfermos en la España medieval*. Barcelona: Península, 2001.

García Icazbalceta, Joaquín. *Bibliografía mexicana del siglo XVI*. Ed. Agustín Millares Carlo. Mexico: Fondo de Cultura Económica, 1954.

García Márquez, Gabriel. 'La soledad de América Latina'. Nobel Lecture. The Nobel Foundation. 1982. www.nobelprize.org/prizes/literature/1982/marquez/lecture/. 30 Apr. 2019.

Garcilaso de la Vega, Inca. *Comentarios reales. La Florida del Inca*. [1609. 1605]. Ed. Mercedes López-Baralt. Madrid: Espasa Calpe, S. A., 2003.

Gómez de Silva, Guido. *Diccionario breve de mexicanismos*. 'aguacate'. 2nd printing. Mexico: Fondo de Cultura Económica, 2004. 6.

Góngora, Luis de. *Poesía selecta*. Eds. Antonio Pérez Lasheras and José María Micó. Madrid: Clásicos Taurus, 1991.

González Sánchez, Carlos Alberto. *New World Literacy: Writing and Culture Across the Atlantic, 1500–1700*. Tr. Tristan Platt. Lewisburg, PN: Bucknell, 2011.

Goodman, David. 'Science, Medicine, and Technology in Colonial Spanish America: New Interpretations, New Approaches'. *Science in the Spanish and Portuguese Empires, 1500–1800*. Eds. Daniela Bleichmar, Paula de Vos, Kristin Huffine and Kevin Sheehan. Stanford, CA: Stanford UP, 2009. 9–34.

Gradie, Charlotte M. 'Discovering the Chichimecas'. *The Americas* 51.1 (1994): 67–88.

Green, Monica H. Ed. and tr. *The Trotula: An English Translation of the Medieval Compendium of Women's Medicine*. Philadelphia: U of Pennsylvania P, 2002.

Hampe Martínez, Teodoro. 'La historiografía el libro en América hispana: un estado de la cuestión'. *Leer en tiempos de la colonia: imprenta, bibliotecas y lectores en la Nueva España*. Eds. Idalia García Aguilar and Pedro Rueda Ramírez. Mexico: UNAM, 2010. 55–72.

Harris, Jonathan Gil. *Foreign Bodies and the Body Politic: Discourses on Social Pathology in Early Modern England*. Cambridge: Cambridge UP, 1998.

Heng, Geraldine. 'Jews, Saracens, "Black Men", Tartars: England in a World of Racial Difference'. *A Companion to Medieval English Literature and Culture, c. 1350–c. 1500*. Ed. Peter Brown. Malden, MA: Blackwell, 2007.

Hernández, Francisco. *Quatro libros de la naturaleza, y virtudes de las plantas, y animales que estan receuidos en el vso de Medicina en la Nueva España, y la Methodo, y correccion, y preparacion, quepara administrallas se requiere con lo que el Doctor Francisco Hernandez escriuio en lengua Latina*. Trad. Francisco Ximénez. Mexico: casa de la Viuda de Diego Lopez Daualos, 1615.

——. *The Mexican treasury: the writings of Dr. Francisco Hernández*. Ed. Simon Varey. Trs. Rafael Chabrán, Cynthia L. Chamberlin and Simon Varey. Stanford, CA: Stanford UP, 2000.

Hernández González, Miguel and José Luis Prieto Pérez. *Historia de la ciencia*. Vol. I. La Orotava, Tenerife: Fundación Canaria Orotava de Historia de la Ciencia, 2007.

Herzog, Tamar. 'Beyond Race: Exclusion in Early Modern Spain and Spanish America'. *Race and Blood in the Iberian World*. Eds. Max S. Hering Torres, María Elena Martínez and David Nirenberg. Zurich, Berlin: LIT Verlag, 2012. 151–67.

Hill, Ruth. 'The Blood of Others: Breeding Plants, Animals, and White People in the Spanish Atlantic'. *The Cultural Politics of Blood, 1500–1900*. Eds. Kimberly Coles, R. Bauer, Z. Nunes and C. L. Peterson. New York: Palgrave Macmillan, 2015. 45–64.

Hill Boone, Elizabeth and Walter Mignolo. Eds. *Writing Without Words: Alternative Literacies in Mesoamerica and the Andes*. Durham, NC: Duke UP, 1994.

Hogarth, Rana A. *Medicalizing Blackness: Making Racial Difference in the Atlantic World, 1780–1840*. Chapel Hill: U of North Carolina P, 2017.

Houdt, Toon Van. 'Lessius's Views on Taxation and Justice: Scholastic Background and Humanist Applications'. *Forms of the 'Medieval' in the 'Renaissance'*. Ed. George Hugo Tucker. Charlottesville, VA: Rookwood Press, 2000. 91–120.

Huarte de San Juan, Juan. *Examen de ingenios*. [1575]. Ed. Guillermo Serrés. Madrid: Cátedra, 1989.

'Inventario de bienes del Inca Garcilaso de la Vega [Archivo de Protocolos de Córdoba, oficio 29, protocolo 35, ff. 521v–525v]'. Transcript by Rosario Navarro Gala. *La biblioteca del Inca Garcilaso de la Vega [1616–2016]*. Madrid: Biblioteca Nacional de España, 2016. 183–97.

Juárez-Almendros, Encarnación. *Disabled Bodies in Early Modern Spanish Literature*. Liverpool: Liverpool UP, 2017.

Kusukawa, Sachiko. *Picturing the Book of Nature: Image, Text and Argument in Sixteenth-Century Human Anatomy and Medical Botany*. Chicago, IL: U of Chicago P, 2012.

Laqueur, Thomas. *Making Sex: Body and Gender from the Greeks to Freud*. Cambridge, MA and London: Harvard UP, 1990.

Ledezma, Domingo. 'Historia natural y discurso idiosincrático del Nuevo Mundo: Los Problemas y secretos maravillosos de las Indias de Juan de Cárdenas (1591)'. *Colorado Review of Hispanic Studies* 7 (Fall 2009): 151–67.

León, Nicolás. Introduction. *Cuatro libros de la naturaleza y virtudes medicinales de las plantas y animales de la Nueva España. Extracto de las obras del Dr Francisco Hernández* (1615). By Francisco Hernández. Tr. Francisco Ximénez. Morelia: Escuela de Artes á cargo de José Rosario Bravo, 1888. v–xxviii.

Leonard, Irving A. *Books of the Brave: Being an Account of Books and of Men in the Spanish Conquest and Settlement of the Sixteenth-Century*. 2nd printing. Berkeley: U of California P, 1992.

Leong, Elaine and Alisha Rankin, 'Introduction: Secrets and Knowledge'. *Secrets and Knowledge in Medicine and Science*, 1500–1800. Eds. Elaine Leong and Alisha Rankin. Surrey: Ashgate, 2011. 1–20.

López Beltrán, Carlos. 'Hippocratic Bodies. Temperament and Castas in Spanish America (1570–1820)'. *Journal of Spanish Cultural Studies* 8.2 (2007): 253–89.

López de Gómara, Francisco. *Historia de Mexico, con el descvbrimiento dela nueua España, conquistada por el muy ilustre y valeroso Principe don Fernando Cortes, Marques del Valle*. Antwerp: Juan Steelsio, 1554.

López de Hinojosos, Alonso. *Suma y Recopilación de Cirugía con un arte para sangrar muy útil y provechosa*. [1578]. Mexico: Academia Nacional de Medicina, 1977.

——. *Svmma, y recopilacion de chirvgia, con vn Arte para sangrar muy vtil y prouechosa*. Mexico: Antonio Ricardo, 1578.

——. *Svmma y recopilacion de cirvgia, con vn arte para sangrar, y examen de barberos*. Mexico: Pedro Balli, 1595.

López de Velasco, Juan. *Geografía y descripción universal de las Indias*. [1574]. Ed. Marcos Jiménez de la Espada. Biblioteca de autores españoles. Vol. 248. Madrid: Ediciones Atlas, 1971.

López Medel, Tomás. *Colonización de América: informes y testimonios, 1549–1572*. Eds. L. Pereña, C. Baciero and F. Maseda. Madrid: Consejo Superior de Investigaciones Científicas, 1990.

López Parada, Esperanza, Marta Ortiz Canseco and Paul Firbas. 'Selección de piezas comentadas'. *La biblioteca del Inca Garcilaso de la Vega [1616–2016]*. Madrid: Biblioteca Nacional de España, 2016. 93–179.

López Piñero, José María. 'El Renacimiento'. *Antología de clásicos médicos*. Madrid: Editorial Tricastela, 1998. 129–37.

——. 'La disección y el saber anatómico en la España de la primera mitad del siglo XVI'. *Cuadernos de Historia de la Medicina Española* 13 (1974): 51–110.

López Piñero, José M., José Luis Fresquet Febrer, María Luz López-Terrada and José Pardo Tomás. *Medicinas, drogas y alimentos vegetales del nuevo mundo: textos e imágenes españolas que los introdujeron en Europa*. Madrid: Ministerio de Sanidad y Consumo, 1992.

López Piñero, José M. and María Luz López-Terrada. *La influencia española en la introducción en Europa de las plantas americanas (1493–1623)*. Cuadernos Valencianos de Historia de la Medicina y la Ciencia. 53. Valencia: Instituto de Estudios Documentales e Históricos sobre la Ciencia, Universitat de València – C.S.I.C., 1997.

——. 'Los primeros libros de medicina impresos en América'. *Viejo y nuevo continente: la medicina en el encuentro de dos mundos*. Ed. José M. López Piñero. Madrid: Saned, 1992. 168–92.

López-Terrada, María Luz. '"Sallow-Faced Girl, Either It's Love or You've Been Eating Clay": The Representation of Illness in Golden Age Theater'. *Medical Cultures of the Early Modern Spanish Empire.* Eds. John Slater, María Luz López-Terrada and José Pardo Tomás. Surrey: Ashgate, 2014. 167–87.

McDougall, Sara. 'Women and Gender in Canon Law'. *The Oxford Handbook of Women and Gender in Medieval Europe.* Eds. Judith M. Bennett and Ruth Mazo Karras. Oxford: Oxford UP, 2013. 163–78.

McVaugh, Michael R. Introduction. *Inventarium sive Chirurgia Magna.* By Guy de Chauliac. [1363]. Ed. and tr. Michael R. McVaugh. Vol. 1. Leiden: E. J. Brill, 1997. ix–xviii.

Marroquín Arredondo, Jaime. 'The Method of Francisco Hernández: Early Modern Science and the Translation of Mesoamerica's Natural History'. *Translating Nature: Cross-Cultural Histories of Early Modern Science.* Eds. Jaime Marroquín Arredondo and Ralph Bauer. Philadelphia: U of Pennsylvania P, 2019. 45–69.

Martínez, María Elena. *Genealogical Fictions: Limpieza de Sangre, Religion, and Gender in Colonial Mexico.* Stanford, CA: Stanford UP, 2008.

——. 'Sex and the Colonial Archive: The Case of "Mariano" Aguilera'. *Hispanic American Historical Review,* 96.3 (2016): 421–43.

——. 'The Black Blood of New Spain: *Limpieza de Sangre,* Racial Violence, and Gendered Power in Early Colonial Mexico'. *The William and Mary Quarterly,* Third Series, 61.3 (2004): 479–520.

Martínez Hernández, Gerardo. 'Limpieza de sangre del doctor Juan de la Fuente, primer catedrático de medicina de la Real Universidad de México (1572)'. *Estudios de Historia Novohispana* 50 (2014): 175–211.

Martínez-San Miguel, Yolanda. *From Lack to Excess: 'Minor' Readings of Latin American Colonial Discourse.* Lewisburg, PN: Bucknell UP, 2008.

Maza, Francisco de la. *Sor Juana Inés de la Cruz ante la historia.* Mexico: Universidad Nacional Autónoma de México, 1980.

Merrim, Stephanie. 'Hispanic New World historiography'. *The Cambridge History of Latin American Literature.* Vol. 1. Cambridge: Cambridge UP, 1996. 58–100.

——. *The Spectacular City, Mexico and Hispanic Literary Culture.* Austin: U of Texas P, 2010.

Mignolo, Walter D. *The Darker Side of the Renaissance: Literacy, Territoriality & Colonization.* 2nd ed. Ann Arbor: U of Michigan P, 2003.

Miguel Alonso, Aurora. 'Las ediciones de la obra de Dioscórides en el siglo XVI. Fuentes textuales e iconográficas'. Alicante: Biblioteca Virtual Miguel de Cervantes, 2008. www.cervantesvirtual.com/obra-visor/las-ediciones-de-la-obra-de-dioscrides-en-el-siglo-xvi-fuentes-textuales-e-iconogrficas-0/html/01e3c7ec-82b2-11df-acc7-002185ce6064_5.html. 13 Jan. 2020.

Millones Figueroa, Luis. 'Filosofía e historia natural en el Inca Garcilaso'. Alicante: Biblioteca Virtual Miguel de Cervantes, 2009. www.cervantes-virtual.com/obra-visor/filosofa-e-historia-natural-en-el-inca-garcilaso-0/html/02426810-82b2-11df-acc7-002185ce6064_2.html#I_0_. 13 Jan. 2020.

——. 'Indianos problemas: la historia natural del doctor Juan de Cárdenas'. *Élites intelectuales y modelos colectivos: mundo ibérico (siglos XVI–XIX).* Madrid: Consejo Superior de Investigaciones Científicas, 2002. 83–100.

Monardes, Nicolás. *Dos libros. El uno trata de todas las cosas que traen de nuestras Indias Occidentales, que sirven al uso de Medicina, y como se ha de usar de la rayz del Mechoacan, purga excelentissima. El otro libro, trata de dos medicinas maravillosas que son contra todo Veneno, la piedra Bezaar, y la yerva Escuençonera. Con la cura de los Venenados. Do veran muchos secretos de naturaleza y de medicina, con grandes experiencias.* Seville: Sebastián Trujillo, 1565.

——. *Segunda parte del libro de las cosas que se traen de nuestras Indias Occidentales, que sirven al uso de medicina.* Seville: Alonso Escrivano, 1571.

Morel-Fatio, Alfred. 'Comer barro'. *Mélanges de Philologie Romane dédiés a Carl Wahlund.* Geneva: Slatkine Reprints, 1972. 41–49.

Mundy, Barbara E. *The Death of Aztec Tenochtitlan, the Life of Mexico City.* Austin: U of Texas P, 2015.

Muñoz Buendía, Antonio. 'Los alumbres de Rodalquilar (Almería): sueños y fracasos de una gran empresa minera del siglo XVI'. *Los señoríos en la Andalucía Moderna. El Marquesado de los Vélez.* Eds. Francisco Andújar Castillo and Julián Pablo Díaz López. Almeria: Instituto de Estudios Almerinenses, 2007. 463–90.

Muriel, Josefina. *Hospitales de la Nueva España. Vol. I. Fundaciones del siglo XVI.* 2nd ed. Mexico: UNAM, Instituto de Investigaciones Históricas and Cruz Roja Mexicana, 1990.

Navarro, Víctor. 'Tradition and Scientific Change in Early Modern Spain: The Role of the Jesuits'. *Jesuit Science and the Republic of Letters.* Ed. Mordechai Feingold. Cambridge, MA & London: MIT UP, 2003. 321–87.

Nemser, Daniel. *Infrastructures of Race: Concentration and Biopolitics in Colonial Mexico.* Austin: U of Texas P, 2017.

Nesvig, Martin Austin. '"Heretical Plagues" and Censorship Cordons: Colonial Mexico and the Transatlantic Book Trade'. *Church History* 75.1 (2006): 1–37.

Ngou-Mve, Nicolás. 'Los orígenes de las rebeliones negras en el México colonial'. *Dimensión antropológica* 6.16 (1999): 7–40.

Norton, Marcy. *Sacred Gifts, Profane Pleasures: A History of Tobacco and Chocolate in the Atlantic World.* Ithaca, NY and London: Cornell UP, 2008.

Núñez, Francisco. *Libro intitvlado del parto humano, en el qual se contienen remedios muy vtiles y vsuales para el parto difficultoso delas mugeres, con otros muchos secretos a ello pertenecientes.* Alcala: Casa de Iuan Gracian, 1580.

OED. *OED Online.* 'scientist, n'. Oxford UP, June 2016. www.oed.com/. 1 Aug. 2016.

Ong, Walter J. 'Commonplace rhapsody: Ravisius Textor, Zwinger and Shakespeare'. *Classical Influences on European Culture A.D. 1500–1700.* Ed. R. R. Bolgar. Cambridge: Cambridge UP, 1976. 91–126.

Orella, José Luis. 'El pensamiento filosófico y médico de Huarte de San Juan'. *Sancho el sabio: revista de cultura e investigación vasca* 6.6 (1996): 49–67.

Pardo Tomás, José. 'Anatomías del Nuevo Mundo: Saberes y prácticas anatómicas en Nueva España en el siglo XVI'. *Ciencia y cultura entre dos mundos. Segundo Simposio. Fuentes documentales y sus diversas interpretaciones.* Eds. José L. Montesinos Sierra and Sergio Toledo Prats. La Orotava: Fundación Canaria Orotava de Historia de la Ciencia, 2011a. 129–55.

——. *El tesoro natural de América. Colonialismo y ciencia en el siglo XVI.* Madrid: Nivola, 2002.

——. 'Natural knowledge and medical remedies in the book of secrets: uses and appropriations in Juan de Cárdenas' *Problemas y secretos maravillosos de las Indias* (Mexico, 1591)'. *A Passion for Plants: Materia Medica and Botany in Scientific Networks from the 16th to the 18th Centuries.* Eds. Sabine Anagnostou, Florike Egmond and Christoph Friedrich. Stuttgart: Wissenschaftliche Verlagsgesellschaft, 2011b. 1–16.

Park, Katharine. 'Cadden, Laqueur, and the "One-Sex Body"'. *Medieval Feminist Forum* 46.1 (2010): 96–100.

——. *Secrets of Women: Gender, Generation, and the Origins of Human Dissection.* New York: Zone Books, 2006.

Park, Katharine and Robert A. Nye. 'Destiny Is Anatomy'. Review of *Making Sex: Body and Gender from the Greeks to Freud.* By Thomas Laqueur. *New Republic* 18 Feb. 1991: 53–57.

Pérez Marín, Yarí. *'Curiosos romancistas': la epistemología europea y la literatura médica novohispana, 1565–1592.* PhD dissertation. Brown University. Ann Arbor: ProQuest/UMI, 2006. (Publication No. AAT 3227901.)

——. 'Empathy, Patients' Needs and Therapeutic Innovation in the Medical Literature of Early Viceregal Mexico'. *Geopolitics, Culture and the Scientific Imaginary in Latin America.* Eds. Joanna Page and María del Pilar Blanco. Gainesville: UP of Florida, 2020. 103–16.

——. 'La tierra enferma: representaciones tempranas del Caribe y el discurso patológico'. *Estudios: Revista de Investigaciones Literarias y Culturales* 17.2 (2009 [2011]): 261–85.

——. 'Medicina e historia natural en los *Comentarios reales* de Inca Garcilaso'. Jornadas Internacionales: Las Indias y los discursos virreinales, Universidad de La Laguna, La Laguna. 16 April 2015. Conference presentation.

——. 'Sound, scale and animal-human distress in early modern Hispanic medical writing'. University of St Andrews, St Andrews. Medicine, Literature and Culture in the Early Modern Hispanic World Conference. 5 July 2017. Conference presentation.

——. 'Suspect Ailments: Illness and Moral Weakness in Late Sixteenth Century New Spain Writings on Women'. *Cincinnati Romance Review* 22 (2003): 148–58.

——. 'The local doctor? Medical writing in Mexico from 1578–1610'. Queen's University, Belfast. The Paths of Medical Un/Orthodoxy? Colonial Latin America and its World Symposium. 9 November 2013. Conference presentation.

Pérez Pascual, José I. 'Algunas aportaciones de la *Suma de la Flor de Cirugía* al conocimiento del léxico medieval castellano'. *Estudios filológicos en homenaje a Eugenio Bustos de Tovar.* Eds. José Antonio Bartol Hernández, Juan Felipe García Santos and Javier de Santiago Guervós. Vol. 2. Salamanca: Ediciones Universidad de Salamanca, 1992. 749–60.

Perromat Augustín, Kevin. *El plagio en las literaturas hispánicas: Historia, Teoría y Práctica.* PhD dissertation. Université Paris-Sorbonne, 2010.

Plato. *The Timaeus and the Critias or Atlanticus.* Tr. Thomas Taylor. Washington, DC: Pantheon Books, 1955.

Porter, Martin. *Windows of the Soul: Physiognomy in European Culture 1470–1780*. Oxford: Oxford UP, 2005.

primeroslibros.org. *Primeros Libros de las Américas: Impresos Americanos del siglo XVI en las Bibliotecas del Mundo*. http://primeroslibros.org/index.html. 16 Sep. 2020.

Rama, Ángel. *La ciudad letrada*. Hanover: Ediciones del Norte, 1984.

Ramírez Santacruz, Francisco. *El diagnóstico de la humanidad por Mateo Alemán: el discurso médico del Guzmán de Alfarache*. Potomac: Scripta Humanistica, 2005.

Rappaport, Joanne and Tom Cummins. *Beyond the Lettered City: Indigenous Literacies in the Andes*. Durham, NC: Duke UP, 2011.

Reyes, Alfonso. 'Notas sobre la inteligencia americana'. *El ensayo mexicano moderno*. Ed. José Luis Martínez. Mexico: Fondo de Cultura Económica, 1958. 302–11.

Risse, Guenter B. 'Shelter and Care for Natives and Colonists: Hospitals in Sixteenth-Century New Spain'. *Searching for the Secrets of Nature: The Life and Works of Dr. Francisco Hernández*. Eds. Simon Varey, Rafael Chabrán and Dora B. Weiner. Stanford, CA: Stanford UP, 2000.

Rodríguez López, Jesús. *Supersticiones de Galicia*. 2nd ed. Madrid: Imprenta de Ricardo Rojas, 1910.

Rodríguez-Sala, María Luisa, Verónica Ramírez, Alfonso Pérez, María de Jesús Ángel and Cecilia Rivera. *El Hospital Real de los Naturales, sus administradores y sus cirujanos (1531–1764) miembros de un estamento ocupacional o de una comunidad científica?* Mexico: UNAM, Academia Mexicana de Cirugía, Patronato del Hospital de Jesús and Secretaría de Salubridad y Asistencia, 2005a.

——. *Los cirujanos de hospitales de la Nueva España (siglos XVI y XVII) ¿miembros de un estamento profesional o de una comunidad científica?*. Mexico: UNAM, Academia Mexicana de Cirugía, Patronato del Hospital de Jesús and Secretaría de Salubridad y Asistencia, 2005b.

Russo, Alessandra. '"Everywhere in this New Spain": Extension and Articulation of an Artistic World'. *Source: Notes in the History of Art* 29.3 (2010): 12–17.

Sabuco de Nantes Barrera, Oliva. *New Philosophy of Human Nature*. [1587]. Ed. and tr. Mary Ellen Waithe, Maria Colomer Vintró and C. Angel Zorita. Urbana and Chicago: U of Illinois P, 2007.

——. *Nveva filosofia dela naturaleza del hombre, no conocida ni alcançada de los grandes filosofos antiguos: la qual mejora la vida y salud humana*. Madrid: P. Madrigal, 1587.

——. *The True Medicine*. [1587]. Ed. and tr. Gianna Pomata. Toronto: Iter, Inc and Centre for Reformation and Renaissance Studies, 2010.

Sagarzazu, María Elvira. '*Baquiano*, un enigma con historia'. *Sharq al-Andalus* 18 (2003–07): 113–29.

Schwaller, Robert C. *Géneros de Gente in Early Colonial Mexico: Defining Racial Difference*. Norman: U of Oklahoma P, 2006.

Shakespeare, William. *The Oxford Shakespeare. The Complete Works*. Eds. John Jowett, William Montgomery, Gary Taylor and Stanley Wells. Oxford and New York: Oxford UP, 2005.

Shapin, Steven. *The Scientific Revolution*. 2nd ed. Chicago, IL and London: U of Chicago P, 2018.

Sherman, William H. *Used Books: Marking Readers in Renaissance England.* Philadelphia: U of Pennsylvania P, 2008.

Shotwell, R. Allen. 'The Revival of Vivisection in the Sixteenth Century'. *Journal of the History of Biology* 46 (2013): 171–97.

Silverblatt, Irene. Foreword. *Imperial Subjects: Race and Identity in Colonial Latin America.* Eds. Andrew B. Fisher and Matthew D. O'Hara. Durham, NC and London: Duke UP, 2009. ix–xii.

Siraisi, Nancy G. *Medieval & Early Renaissance Medicine: An Introduction to Knowledge and Practice.* Chicago, IL: U of Chicago P, 1990.

Skaarup, Bjørn Okholm. *Anatomy and Anatomists in Early Modern Spain.* Farnham: Ashgate, 2015.

Skinner, Patricia. 'Marking the Face, Curing the Soul? Reading the Disfigurement of Women in the Later Middle Ages'. *Medicine, Religions and Gender in Medieval Culture.* Ed. Naoë Kukita Yoshikawa. Suffolk: Boydell & Brewer Ltd, 2015. 181–201.

Slisco, Aila. 'GOP senator defends "Chinese virus" name, says it's not racist because China is where "these viruses emanate from"'. *Newsweek* 18 March 2020: n. pag. *Newsweek.com.* www.newsweek.com/gop-senator-defends-chinese-virus-name-says-its-not-racist-because-china-where-these-viruses-1493145. 23 March 2020.

Socolow, Susan Migden. *The Women of Colonial Latin America.* 2nd ed. Cambridge: Cambridge UP, 2014.

Solomon, Michael. *Fictions of Well-Being: Sickly Readers and Vernacular Medical Writing in Late Medieval and Early Modern Spain.* Philadelphia: U of Pennsylvania P, 2010.

——. 'Women Healers and the Power to Disease in Late Medieval Spain'. *Women Healers and Physicians: Climbing a Long Hill.* Lexington: UP of Kentucky, 1997. 79–92.

Somolinos d'Ardois, Germán. 'Relación alfabética de los profesionistas médicos, o en conexión con la medicina, que practicaron en territorio mexicano (1521–1618)'. *Capítulos de historia médica mexicana.* Vol. 3. Mexico: Sociedad Mexicana de Historia y Filosofía de la Medicina, 1980a.

——. 'Relación y estudio de los impresos médicos mexicanos redactados y editados desde 1521 a 1618'. *Capítulos de la historia médica mexicana.* Vol. 4. Mexico: Sociedad Mexicana de Historia y Filosofía de la Medicina, 1980b.

——. 'Vida y obra de Alonso López de Hinojosos'. *Suma y recopilación de cirugía con un arte para sangrar muy útil y provechosa.* By Alonso López de Hinojosos. Mexico: Academia Nacional de Medicina, 1977. 1–46.

Stone, Erin. 'Chasing "Caribs": Defining Zones of Legal Indigenous Enslavement in the Circum-Caribbean, 1493–1542'. *Slaving Zones: Cultural Identities, Ideologies, and Institutions in the Evolution of Global Slavery.* Eds. Jeff Fynn-Paul and Damian Alan Pargas. Leiden: Brill, 2018. 118–47.

Surtz, Ronald E. 'Botanical and Racial Hybridity in the *Comentarios reales* of El Inca Garcilaso'. *Mediterranean Identities in the Premodern Era: Entrepôts, Islands, Empires.* Eds. John Watkins and Kathryn L. Reyerson. Farnham, Surrey: Ashgate Publishing Limited, 2014. 249–63.

Sweet, James H. 'The Iberian Roots of American Racist Thought'. *The William and Mary Quarterly*, 3rd Series 54.1 (1997): 143–66.

Taylor-Pearce, Deborah. 'Portraits of Melancholy Gallery Exhibit, III: Cavendish's "Studious She is and all Alone" frontispiece, 1655'. *She-philospher.com*. 18 Aug. 2007. https://she-philosopher.com/gallery/melancholyP3.html. 3 Apr. 2020.

Tenorio, Martha Lilia. 'La función social de la lengua poética en el virreinato'. *Historia sociolingüística de México*. Vol. 1. Eds. Rebeca Barriga Villanueva and Pedro Martín Butragueño. Mexico: Colegio de México, 2010. 347–402.

Trabulse, Elías. *Los orígenes de la ciencia moderna en México (1630–1680)*. Mexico: Fondo de Cultura Económica, 1994.

Tortorici, Zeb. 'Introduction: Unnatural Bodies, Desires and Devotions'. In *Sexuality and the Unnatural in Colonial Latin America*. Ed. Zeb Tortorici. Oakland: U of California P, 2016. 1–22.

——. *Sins against Nature: Sex and Archives in Colonial New Spain*. Durham, NC: Duke UP, 2018.

Twinam, Ann. *Purchasing Whiteness: Pardos, Mulattos, and the Quest for Social Mobility in the Spanish Indies*. Stanford, CA: Stanford UP, 2015.

Uranga, Emilio. 'El doctor Juan de Cárdenas (1563–1609): su vida y obra'. *Memorias del Primer Coloquio Mexicano de Historia de la Ciencia*. Vol. 1. Mexico: Sociedad Mexicana de Historia Natural, 1964. 71–110.

——. 'Juan de Cárdenas: sus amigos y sus enemigos'. *Historia de la ciencia y la tecnología*. Ed. Elías Trabulse. Mexico: Colegio de México, 1991. 37–58.

U.S. National Library of Medicine. *Historical Anatomies on the Web*. U.S. National Library of Medicine. 2003. https://www.nlm.nih.gov/exhibition/historicalanatomies/home.html. 9 Aug. 2020.

Vågene, Åshild. J., Alexander Herbig, Michael G. Campana, Nelly M. Robles García, Christina Warinner, Susanna Sabin, Maria A. Spyrou, Aida Andrades Valtueña, Daniel Huson, Noreen Tuross, Kirsten I. Bos and Johannes Krause. '*Salmonella enterica* genomes from victims of a major sixteenth-century epidemic in Mexico'. *Nature Ecology & Evolution*, Vol. 2 (March 2018): 520–28.

Van Deusen, Nancy E. *Global Indios: The Indigenous Struggle for Justice in Sixteenth-Century Spain*. Durham, NC: Duke UP, 2015.

Velasco, Sherry. *Male Delivery: Reproduction, Effeminacy, and Pregnant Men in Early Modern Spain*. Nashville, TN: Vanderbilt UP, 2016.

Vesalius, Andreas. *On the Fabric of the Human Body. Book I: The Bones and Cartilages*. [De Humani Corporis Fabrica Libri Septem]. Trs. William Frank Richardson and John Burd Carman. San Francisco, CA: Norman Publishing, 1998.

Viesca-Treviño, Carlos and Patricia Aceves-Pastrana. 'Juan de la Fuente, primer catedrático de medicina en la Real y Pontificia Universidad de México'. *Revista Médica del Instituto Mexicano del Seguro Social* 49.4 (2011): 451–58.

Villaseñor Black, Charlene. 'Portraits of Sor Juana Inés de la Cruz and the Dangers of Intellectual Desire'. *Sor Juana Inés de la Cruz: Selected Works*. Ed. Anna More. New York: W. W. Norton & Co, 2016. 213–30.

Virués Ortega, Javier, Gualberto Buela-Casal and Heliodoro Carpintero Capell. 'Una aproximación a la vida de Juan Huarte de San Juan: los primeros años de práctica profesional (1560–1578)'. *Psicothema* 28.2 (2006): 232–37.

Wade, Peter. *Degrees of Mixture, Degrees of Freedom: Genomics, Multiculturalism, and Race in Latin America*. Durham, NC: Duke UP, 2017.

Zamora, Margarita. *Language, Authority, and Indigenous History in the Comentarios reales de los Incas*. Cambridge: Cambridge UP, 1988.

Županov, Ines G. '"The Wheel of Torments": mobility and redemption in Portuguese colonial India (sixteenth century)'. *Cultural Mobility: A Manifesto*. Ed. Stephen Greenblatt. Cambridge: Cambridge UP, 2010. 24–74.

Index

Printed and bound by CPI Group (UK) Ltd, Croydon, CR0 4YY

13/09/2026

14961097-0003